Making Vegan Meat

Making Vegan Meat

THE PLANT-BASED FOOD SCIENCE COOKBOOK

MARK THOMPSON

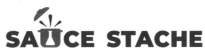

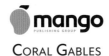

mango

PUBLISHING GROUP

CORAL GABLES

Cover Design: Morgane Leoni
Cover/Interior Photos: © Mark Lee Thompson
Art Direction: Morgane Leoni
Photography: p.44 © beats_ | p.66 © 5ph | stock.adobe.com

For permission requests, please contact the publisher at:
Mango Publishing Group
2850 S Douglas Road, 2nd Floor
Coral Gables, FL 33134 USA
info@mango.bz

For special orders, quantity sales, course adoptions and corporate sales, please email the publisher at sales@mango.bz. For trade and wholesale sales, please contact Ingram Publisher Services at customer.service@ingramcontent.com or +1.800.509.4887.

Making Vegan Meat: The Plant-Based Food Science Cookbook

Library of Congress Cataloging-in-Publication number: 2021936138
ISBN: (print) 978-1-64250-600-6, (ebook) 978-1-64250-601-3
BISAC category code HEA017000, HEALTH & FITNESS / Diet & Nutrition / Nutrition

Printed in the United States of America

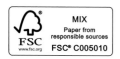

To the love of my life, Monica, for inspiring me,

motivating me, and constantly pushing

me to be a better man, more creative, and for

the idea that started this whole wild journey!

Thank you for roughing it out with me

while this whole thing worked out,

Love you

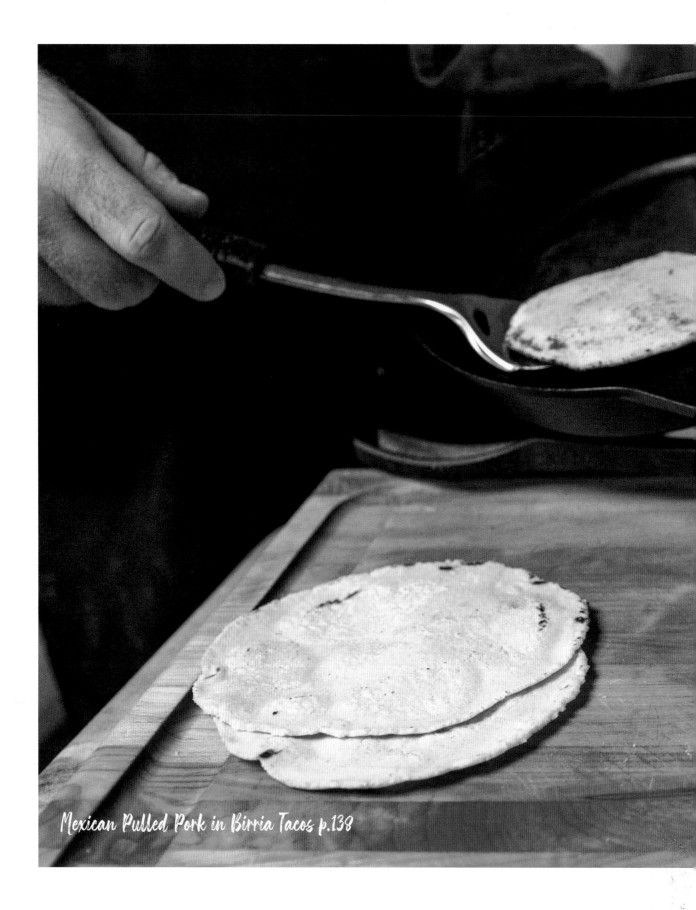

Mexican Pulled Pork in Birria Tacos p.138

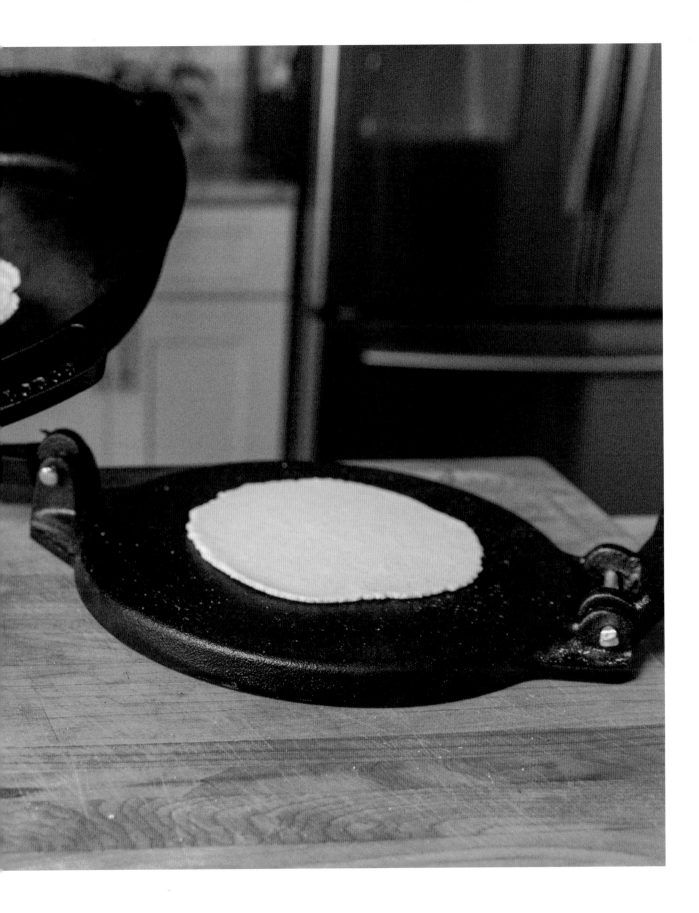

CONTENTS

Vegan
Meat

WHAT EXACTLY IS THIS BOOK?

First... *Look at this!! Look at it!!* It's a cookbook, recipe guide, instruction manual. I wanted to make this book more than just something you pick up from time to time to check out a new recipe—more of a guide into how I make the plant-based meat you see on Sauce Stache. I wanted to give you the insight to how I come up with the flavors, smells, and textures of my recipes, so you can experiment and make your own creations.

When reading this book and working your way through these "recipes," please don't follow them step by step, don't use exactly the same seasonings, sauces, and ingredients that I use. Try something new... *Experiment!* Maybe make something once to see how it comes out, but then next time replace the protein with something completely different—you might be surprised what happens. I want you to find your flavor, find the satisfying texture you're looking for in plant-based meat. For everyone that is different! I realized the things that I enjoyed about the tastes and textures of meat are completely different from what you might enjoy, and that's why this cookbook (guide) will walk you through, not only how to make the creations I make in my kitchen, but exactly what each ingredient is doing there. You might find clues on how you can substitute something to make a recipe even better, you might figure out a way to make something taste exactly like you remember it, you might find a way to nail that perfect taste that'll make anyone's mouth water. I hope you find this cookbook enjoyable on many levels. I hope it feeds, not just your appetite for good food, but also your appetite for creativity.

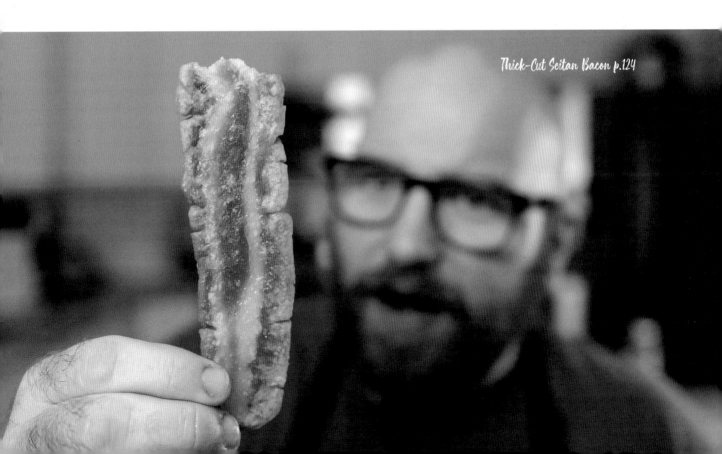

Thick-Cut Seitan Bacon p.124

How Did I End Up Here?

From a young age, I always was interested in how stuff works, how it's made, and how the heck I could make it at home. This was everything from electronics to musical instruments, cars, toys—everything. Needless to say, I took a *lot* of things apart and tried to put them back together. Pair that need to figure things out with a need to create something new, and you end up with Sauce Stache. Sauce Stache started as an outlet for my creativity, and a way to create something fun and interesting. Its original intention was sauce recipes. In early 2016, I started dating Monica, my fiancée. At the time, she ran a yoga blog and YouTube channel. I loved what she did and her passion for creating content and running her own business built around the blog; it was a topic that came up quite early on in our relationship. Sometime near the end of August 2016, Monica said I should make a blog based on my sauce recipes, something I made often when I would cook for our early dates. That blog idea quickly shifted into a YouTube channel. I had fun during the first few months of Sauce Stache—learning how to edit and film videos, buying my first real camera from a pawn shop—but it quickly changed into me wanting to do more. I stepped in front of the camera about nine months later and started making videos about trends, secretly keeping them mostly pescatarian, using vegan products where I could.

Why Plant-Based Food?

I love plant-based food. It opens a whole new world of culinary adventure that you can feel good about and bonus—you get to save animals. Everyone has their own reasons for eating plant-based foods, either health-based, animal-based, environmental-based, all of the above, or a million reasons in between. Making plant-based food is where I can be my most creative, trying new ways, using new techniques, to make food better. I am not trying to reinvent the wheel, just make the wheel taste more like steak than anyone else has. Plant-based diets have been around for a *long* time, all the way back to before 300 BC, and plant-based meat isn't something that's new or trendy. Early vegetarians would boil soy milk to make soy skin, then take that soy skin and tightly pack it together with seasonings and flavors to create a mock meat that had texture and flavors similar to real meat! Plant-based meat has a ton of room for improvement. I want to be a part of this journey and it seems like you do too.

How Do I Use This Cookbook?

I love to find analogies to make things feel easier than they are. This will hopefully be like doing a test backward with all the answers laid out in front of you. Skip the next part, where I explain all the bases, textures, and additives, and how I use them; make some recipes first, figure out what you like and don't like. Do you like the texture of one recipe, but not some of the flavors? Head to the ingredients index on the next few pages and check out the cross-referencing section to see if you can plan a flavor combo that you think you'll like better. Do that over and over again. Then you can start putting together your own creations!

MUST-HAVE INGREDIENTS AND TOOLS

The Pantry: My Favorite Ingredients

Mushrooms are great to have ready in the fridge or dried in the pantry. They can be an awesome protein staple in plant-based meats, the star of any dish. You can essentially make just about anything out of mushrooms, from seafood to pulled pork, or just cook them as mushrooms because they are great how they are.

KING OYSTER MUSHROOM
—

I first came across the king oyster mushroom at my local Asian market. I had never seen a mushroom that big. The king oyster mushroom looks similar to its smaller counterpart, the oyster mushroom, just ten times the size. I first tried this when making mushroom bacon, and I was blown away by its texture and mild but meaty taste. Since then, I have used the king oyster mushroom to make vegan ribs, vegan pulled pork, vegan scallops, and vegan calamari! This is a fun mushroom to experiment with because of its size. You can cut it, slice it, chop it, or cube it. Experiment with it to see what you can come up with.

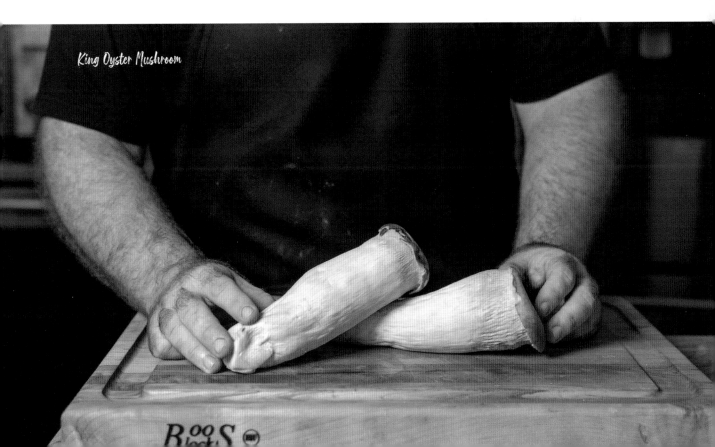

King Oyster Mushroom

PINK OYSTER MUSHROOM

—

The pink oyster mushroom came to me when I was searching for meaty mushrooms. It has this fantastic ability to taste and smell like pork and slightly bacony when pan-fried. Pink oyster mushrooms might be tough to come by in your local stores, but they are very easy to grow on your own using one of the many available grow-at-home kits. You can pan-fry these for little bacon-like chips, season them, press and sear for a more meat-like steak, or simply sauté to add to any dish!

LION'S MANE MUSHROOM

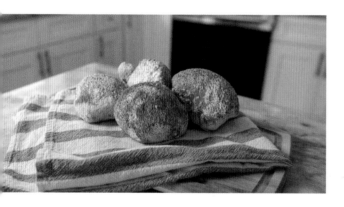

These mushrooms are absolutely incredible and have so many wonderful uses. I first discovered this mushroom after visiting with a local mushroom grower. This mushroom is very easy to grow indoors and is readily available from your local mushroom purveyor. The lion's mane is a large mushroom with what looks like a lion's beard, but is really just spines that grow from the mushroom. This mushroom has a very unique texture that can be pulled apart to mimic crab meat. The really neat thing about this mushroom is that, along with the crab-meat-like texture, it also has a very seafood-like smell and taste. I've pulled these apart to use in crab cakes, but I've also simply sliced them lengthwise to make a lion's mane steak. You can season them with just a touch of salt and pepper, pan-fry, and enjoy. These mushrooms can be found fresh or dried. I can always find dried lions' mane at my local Asian market. Sometimes they go by the name monkey head mushroom.

CHICKEN OF THE WOODS MUSHROOM

—

Chicken of the woods mushrooms are some of my absolute favorite mushrooms. Their texture and taste incredibly resembles chicken! They are very dense and have long strands of textured "meat." The chicken of the woods often gets confused with the hen of the woods, which gets its name simply from looking like a hen, whereas chicken of the woods gets its name because it *tastes just like chicken!* I've pan-fried these, breaded them with eleven herbs and spices, and I've even baked them, and no matter how you prepare them, they always come out with that incredible chicken taste. They are hard to come by, so check online for some mushroom sellers. If you can find them fresh, you are in luck, but they are also available dried.

THE LOBSTER MUSHROOM

—

One of the most flavorful mushrooms on this list, the lobster mushroom gets its name from the fact that it smells, tastes, and kind of looks like lobster. The neat thing about this mushroom is that it actually consists of two different fungi: your basic white mushroom and the red fungus that grows on the outside. I have used this mushroom to make an incredible lobster-like lobster roll simply by frying in butter and then adding all the lobster seasonings you would add (Old bay does a number on this one). Your whole house will be smelling like fresh lobster when you are done cooking this one, so take it all in.

The lobster mushroom is another that is hard to come by. You can find them fresh or dried, usually online. They are only available when they are in season because these mushrooms only grow in nature!

Some of my favorite meaty vegetables and fruits through the years have been those I can find at my local Asian markets. There is always something interesting that my local grocery just doesn't carry. I love to pick up large crazy vegetables, take them home, and figure out what to do with them. I've learned about so many incredible dishes this way and have learned a lot of valuable lessons.

DAIKON RADISH

—

I first stumbled on the daikon at sushi restaurants, but I had no idea what it was. This stringy, crunchy plate dressing was not something that I was really interested in exploring further until I saw it in person. It looks like a giant white carrot...well, sometimes. You can find pretty normal-size daikons around, but most of the time, these things are huge. One of my favorite uses for daikon is to julienne it with some carrots and pickle it. My second favorite use for these monster radishes is to slice them and then flavor them like bacon. This recipe is in the book and is one of my all-time favorite vegan bacon recipes. I love the daikon because of its versatility. It has a nice crunch and a fibrous texture, and easily takes on any flavor you throw at it. I would pick some up, pickle it, chop it, cube it, flavor it, and go to town with it! See what you can come up with using this beautiful blank canvas of a vegetable!

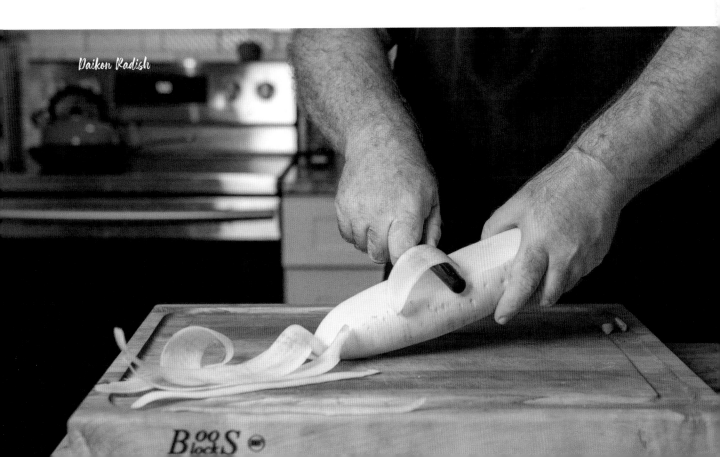

Daikon Radish

WATERMELON RADISH

—

This radish is unique in many ways, but also shares many characteristics with the daikon radish. They both have a very mild peppery taste, a nice blank canvas to start with, but are also very different. The watermelon radish has a wild pink striped color on the inside, and a slightly looser fibrous bite than the daikon radish. I came across this radish after seeing chefs smoking them, then slicing them thin and flavoring them like prosciutto. That was first done by Chef Will Horowitz, the guy who also popularized smoked watermelon ham. One of my favorite things to do with this radish is to brine it in my meaty-flavor broth, then cook it up like beef. You get an incredible texture, like nothing else, that is so meaty you'll think your mind is playing tricks on you.

YOUNG GREEN JACKFRUIT

—

Canned jackfruit should be in every plant-based-meat eater's pantry at all times. This is by far one of the most versatile items on this list, and the possibilities for meaty plants are almost endless here. I have seen so many amazing chefs create incredible dishes using jackfruit, and I have thrown in my creativity a few times on some wild uses for this fruit. You will see it pop up in quite a few recipes in this book. One of the main reasons is because of its incredibly mild texture and taste. Add some chicken flavoring and you have yourself some pulled chicken; add BBQ sauce and you get some really great pulled pork. Ball this up with some binders, flavor it, and deep-fry it, and you get a wild jackfruit nugget. Really, the possibilities are endless. Make sure you check out my jackfruit chicken and waffles or Nashville hot jackfruit. You will not regret it!

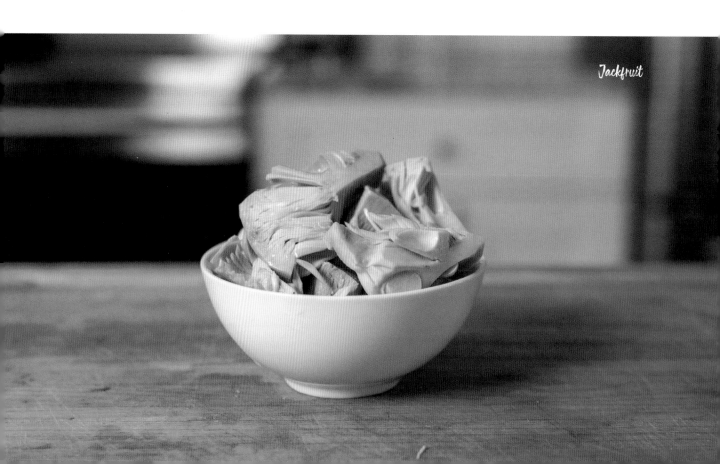

Jackfruit

Now for the rest of my pantry staples. This might feel like we are taking a dive into science class. But don't worry! These are all the same ingredients that can be found in high-end name-brand plant-based foods covering every store shelf. Most of the time I discover these ingredients simply by googling the ingredients labels of my favorite foods. Once you understand what you are eating, you will start to discover new ways of using the same things that are already in your food to make things better.

Binders, Thickeners, and Fillers

METHYLCELLULOSE
—

When I was on my original hunt for a way to recreate those impossibly real plant-based store-bought burgers at home, one ingredient kept popping out at me. Methylcellulose was in everything. I did a little research to see what it did and figure out why it was in just about every plant-based meat product I could find, and I discovered what an incredible ingredient it is. It is a thickener and an emulsifier, and it firms when it is heated and softens when cooled. This process can be repeated multiple times until you reach your desired texture. The more you cook it and cool it, the firmer it gets. For most of my meat recipes, I use a high-viscosity version. I use it in almost all my plant-based meats, and it's a blast to experiment with. It will mix and stay stable with most cold liquids.

KAPPA CARRAGEENAN
—

This gelling hydrocolloid is another thickener and gelling agent. This almost magical ingredient has an incredible firming reaction to a heating and cooling process. Most noticeably used in vegan cheese to help firm the cheese, it still allows the cheese to melt! I've found that kappa carrageenan works wonderfully to create "meat" marbling fat that helps retain textures while also allowing the rendering of the fat as oils. Kappa carrageenan is extracted from a wild red seaweed. You can experiment with this by adding it in small amounts to almost any liquid. It's stable at a neutral pH, meaning if your liquid is too acidic or too alkaline, it won't set properly. If you think your liquid is too acidic, add a pinch of baking soda to make it more neutral.

AGAR AGAR
—

Agar agar is the perfect vegan gelatin substitute. Like kappa carrageenan, agar agar is also extracted from a species of red seaweed. It dissolves in liquid under heat and firms when cooled. It can melt and reset multiple times. It can stay set at a very high temperature, up to around 185°F.

KONJAC GUM
—

This is one of the main ingredients in konnayaku, which is a calorie-free plant-based steak popular in Japan. I first started exploring konjac gum when I was looking into plant-based seafood manufacturing. I found that most seafoods, including shrimp and raw fish, used konjac powder or konjac gum. Konjac has an incredible ability to gel into a fairly solid structure. This reaction happens with the addition of calcium hydroxide, which also helps by adding a slightly fishy taste.

XANTHAN GUM
—

You have probably seen this in grocery stores and on food labels. It is in sauces, soups, cereals, yogurts, cheeses, and drinks. I knew the name well before I ever even thought about what goes into making plant-based meats. It's a thickening agent and stabilizer. If you have a sauce that likes to settle rapidly, add some xanthan gum. Do you want to make a liquid thicker? Use xanthan gum. Want to make a liquid really thick? Use a *lot* of xanthan gum. Xanthan gum also has the unique ability to get thinner when a force is applied and thicken at rest. This works out really well when you're making sauces and you want seasonings to be evenly dispersed without settling, but also want the sauce to thin out when being poured. This thickening and thinning works well when producing an egg-like consistency, and keeps flavor distributed when a product is cooking or setting.

SODIUM ALGINATE
—

This incredible additive has a wild ability to firm in the presence of calcium. Sodium alginate is commonly used for specification. That's where I first saw alginate used but I got excited when I started to see its name pop up in different plant-based products, specifically sausage links. Because of its firming ability with calcium, it works incredibly well to make a skin or a casing over vegan meats or to make tiny liquid-filled orbs like roe or caviar, and I've found great uses for it in seitan to assist with texture!

CALCIUM CHLORIDE/ CALCIUM LACTATE
—

Used as the gelling agent with sodium alginate. Use calcium chloride when alginate is part of your recipe. Calcium chloride is best used when you're not adding calcium to your recipe, as calcium chloride has a bitter taste. Calcium lactate is best used when you are adding calcium to your recipe and alginate is the gelling agent, as in the tomato egg recipe in this book.

TAPIOCA STARCH
—

What an incredible starch this is! Tapioca starch is extracted from the root of the cassava plant. This starch has loads of uses, from pudding, boba pearls, crackers, and candies to baking. Its uses in plant-based meats range from fat binders, creating gels, or as a thickener to create more stable binds in TVP or seitan.

POTATO STARCH
—

Potato starch is such a fun starch to play with. I've recently used it to make bacon, but I've also used it as a binder and thickener. It works well on its own, as it will firm when cooked, but it also has the gelling ability to create a viscous gum.

WHEAT STARCH

—

Wheat starch is the starch from wheat flour. It's also the byproduct of flour-washed seitan. Wheat starch can be used for texture, binding, and as a thickener. In vegan meats, it works very well as a fat substitute.

GLUTINOUS RICE FLOUR

—

I originally used glutinous rice flour when I was attempting to make mochi. Mochi is a chewy rice cake common in Japan. You can find mochi in many variations, but one of the most popular in the US is mochi ice cream. It's sweet mochi wrapped around a ball of ice cream, and it's absolutely delicious. Now, after that introduction, it's probably odd to find it in a book about plant-based meat, but glutinous rice has an incredible stretchy and sticky consistency that works out really well in certain recipes. I've been able to use it successfully in mock fat and plant-based bacon. It's something I am still experimenting with, but I definitely recommend having it in the pantry to play with.

SOY LECITHIN

—

This food additive works great as lubricant and emulsifier. It works great to keep oil emulsifications stable and works well as a filler along with an egg replacer.

ARROWROOT

—

Another starch on the list. Used commonly as a thickener, egg replacer, and binder. Commonly added to vegan cheeses.

CHIA SEEDS/FLAX SEEDS

—

Chia seeds can hold up to ten times their weight in water. They both work great as either a thickener or a gelling agent. Great egg replacer.

VERSAWHIP 600K

—

Versawhip is an egg white replacer. It's a modified soy protein that helps add whipping ability to any nonfat liquid.

Protein Additives and Texture

PEA PROTEIN

—

It would be impossible to write a book about meat without including a protein! Pea protein has been the star child of plant-based meats over the last few years. I originally read about it being used in commercial chicken substitutes, then it made its way into some of my favorite plant burgers. It was extremely difficult to find a pea protein isolate when I originally searched for it, but it has been slowly making its way onto store shelves. I've found pea protein to have a very mild taste and come together well when using binders and thickeners to create additional depth and texture in plant-based meats.

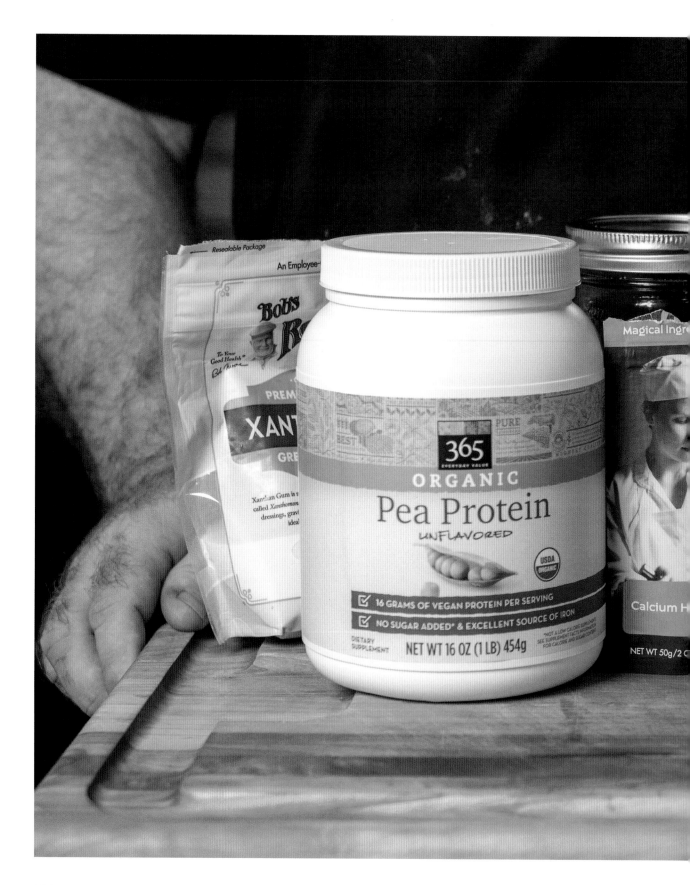

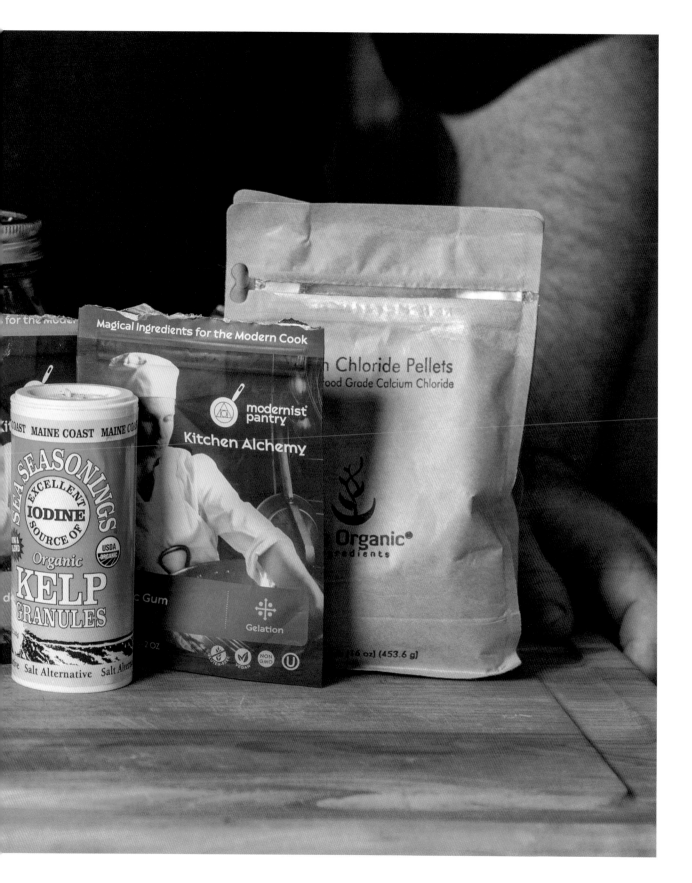

POTATO PROTEIN

—

I recently started using potato protein as a protein filler and egg replacer. I haven't gotten to experiment more with this than making a few eggs, and using it in burgers, but once this product becomes more readily available, I will be testing the heck out of it.

TEXTURED VEGETABLE PROTEIN

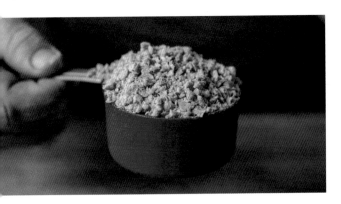

This product has been around for years, and most people have never heard of it, even though they've probably eaten it. Invented by Archer Daniels Midland in the '60s, then used extensively in canned chili as filler, it didn't take long before veggie eaters found it useful for creating incredibly realistic meaty textures. I use TVP in my burger recipes and anywhere I want a ground consistency. It comes in loads of different shapes, including large and small chucks, and is usually not flavored.

VITAL WHEAT GLUTEN

—

One of my favorite texture creators, and one that I'm always trying to replicate. Gluten is a protein of wheat. You can make wheat gluten at home simply by making a dough ball, vigorously kneading it, then washing it, effectively removing the starch. This process develops a really great gluten ball known as seitan. Vital wheat gluten is the already-processed version of that dough ball, dried. You can use it in plant-based meats to add texture. It can be used on its own with water or flavored broth or added to another textured product or vegetable to bind and add texture. Wheat gluten has been used as a meat replacement for thousands of years and is most popular in China and Japan.

Flavor Additives

MUSHROOM EXTRACT SEASONING

—

Every time I visited my local Asian market, I would see a shelf lined with bags of mushroom seasoning. I always assumed it was simply a dried mushroom powder, like what you see on other stores' shelves. Even reading the labels of most of these mushroom seasonings, they usually sounded pretty basic. Dried mushrooms, mushroom extract, and salt. It wasn't until after I finally made the leap to bring some home that I realized the absolute magic that this ingredient is. These packages are secret pouches of umami bombs…little dried nuggets of flavor that pack a punch unlike any seasoning I'd tried before. This has become my go-to when cooking; I sprinkle a pinch of it on everything and load it into most of my plant-based meats. It's always added to my pasta sauces and any gravy. I sprinkle it on my popcorn and French fries, and it's always an addition to any soup or broth I make. This one ingredient will absolutely change the way you season your food.

KELP GRANULES

—

Searching for a fishy flavor, I came across kelp granules. Kelp granules pack a nice fishy flavor in a much smaller package than nori seaweed sheets, and they don't affect the texture. Commonly, in most plant-based seafoods, nori sheets are used to impart the sea flavor. I always had a problem with that simply because they are generally very mild-tasting and have their own texture. Kelp granules are small dissolvable granules of kelp that pack a much bigger punch of flavor. Anytime I want to add a fish-like taste to anything, this is my go-to.

LACTIC ACID

—

One of my star ingredients is lactic acid. I use it any time I want to give something a cheese-like flavor or to increase the acidity of a food. Lactic acid is commonly found in dairy products, but vegan lactic acid is produced from fermented sugar beets. You can add it to tofu and blend to make a sour cream or add a pinch to any vegan cheese recipe to make it even cheesier.

MARMITE/YEAST EXTRACT

—

I was seeing "yeast extract" everywhere in the food industry. A very common form of yeast extract is spent brewer's yeast. The flavor is very meaty. When added to liquid and made into a broth, it can almost perfectly mimic a beef broth. I like to use Marmite, a slightly flavored yeast extract, in just about any "beef" recipe I make.

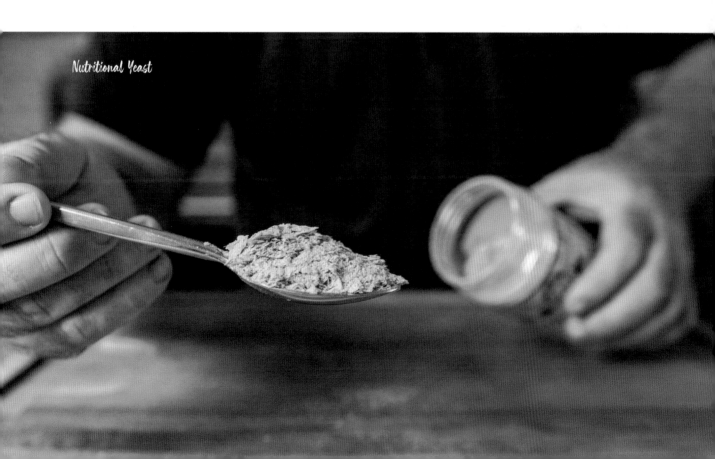

Nutritional Yeast

NUTRITIONAL YEAST

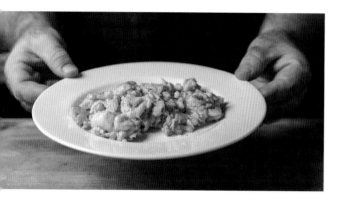

Nutritional yeast, or nooch, is a yeast that is naturally harvested and dried. A dead yeast. This is very different from active dry yeast or baker's yeast. This yeast tastes like cheese. It's the perfect topping on popcorn or fries, but it also goes well in any cheese recipe. Just like its yeast extract friend, it has a very savory flavor. This savory flavor works well in plant-based cheeses, and if flavored right, can also help boost the savories of just about any plant-based meat.

BEETROOT POWDER

Another one of my favorites. Beetroot powder has a unique taste that adds earthiness to just about any recipe. One of my favorite things about it is its color-changing property. Beetroot powder is pink when it's raw, but when it is heated, it turns brown. It's responsible for the fresh raw meat look in my TVP burger and for its ability to brown when cooked and still have a pink center!

More Pantry Items to Consider

VINEGAR POWDER

—

Vinegar, but in a powdered form. When you need the taste, but also need to avoid diluting your mixture.

BOB'S RED MILL EGG REPLACER

—

Great all-around egg replacer.

CANNED CHICKPEAS (AQUAFABA)

—

Aquafaba is the next best egg replacer, and it'll whip into a meringue in no time. Aquafaba can also be used as a binder and is just a good all-around egg replacer to keep canned in the pantry. The best part about needing aquafaba is you'll have a load of chickpeas to use for some hummus!

COCONUT MILK/COCONUT CREAM

—

Both different, both great milk/cream replacements that are great to have in the pantry.

DRIED YUBA/BEAN CURD SHEETS

—

I have a recipe for this, but you can also buy them dried or frozen. They work great in so many recipes for vegan meat skin or to enhance the texture of meat. I also have a bacon made out of these. Super useful.

SHANGGIE BROTH MIX CHICKEN, BEEF, PORK

—

These flavor broth mixes can be found in a lot of Asian markets. If you can't find shanggie, just take a look at the broth mixes in your grocery store. You'll be surprised how many chicken broths don't contain chicken.

MSG

—

Don't hate me for this one, I don't believe the unhealthy hype. MSG is monosodium glutamate, and glutamate is responsible for pretty much all savory flavors. I don't use MSG in the book, but you can substitute it anywhere I used mushroom powder. Just make sure to only use a quarter as much MSG as you would mushroom powder. Pretty much just a tiny pinch will boost the savory in loads of dishes. If a quarter of the amount is more than a teaspoon, then it's too much!

BLACKSTRAP MOLASSES

—

Blackstrap molasses is a dark brown "sludge" that is made in the process of refining sugar. Out of all the molasses stages of processing, it's the last, meaning it's the darkest and sludgy-est. It's also loaded with minerals, including a lot of *iron*. When you want your food to taste meaty, you need *iron*. It's what gives meat the "bloody" taste. That steak taste you might miss? A big part of that is the iron. This is a great one to have in the pantry.

LIQUID SMOKE

—

I just *love* liquid smoke. You'll be able to tell, once you get through a few of my bacon recipes. It just adds this very realistic smoky flavor that I honestly thought you could only get from a massive BBQ pit smoker. It's cheap, and a little goes a long way. Add a bit to just about any recipe to give it that just-off-the-smoker taste.

COCONUT, VEGETABLE, CANOLA, AND OLIVE OILS

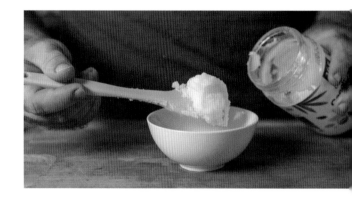

I use coconut oil the most in my recipes. It has a great smoke point, but really has a unique ability to provide fat. Always look for refined coconut oil for any of my recipes, as a non-refined coconut oil will have a coconut taste. I am assuming you don't want your meat to taste like coconut.

I also use canola oil and olive oils throughout the book and on the show. I don't have a preference besides using olive oil for most recipes where the oil is mixed in last or after cooking.

You can also check out algae oil. It has a mild taste and works great to give a fatty feeling to any of the seafood dishes in the book. As always, experiment!

My Favorite Kitchen Tools and Necessities

DOUBLE-SCREW TOFU PRESS

—

This is one of my favorite styles of tofu press because it can be used for so much more than tofu. It looks like two plastic cutting boards with two long screws and two big wing nuts that attach everything together. The great thing about this is that it leaves both sides open, so you can put in larger items that need to be squeezed. I've definitely wrapped seitan in cheesecloth and thrown it at my tofu press to get a denser or chewy texture.

NUT MILK BAG/CLOTH COFFEE FILTER

—

There are so many nut milk bags on the market, it's hard to decide which one is going to work the best as a fine strainer and squeezable pouch to make nut milks, or to strain out and squeeze tofu and other vegan meats. There are so many uses for these bags, beyond coffee filters or nut milk, so these had to go on my list of necessities. My favorites are the Thai tea bags that have a long metal or wood handle at the top.

FOOD DEHYDRATOR

—

When making vegan meats, a lot of times you'll need a dehydrator. A dehydrator works great because it is a tool designed specifically to do one task and do it well. Commonly, when making videos, I tend to stick to using my oven when dehydrating foods because that is the most common appliance in people's households, but off camera I always go straight for my dehydrator. It works quicker than an oven to dehydrate food, but also is more energy-efficient.

FOOD SCALE

—

A food scale is at the top of my priority list for things to have in your kitchen. When experimenting with making any sort of food, having a scale can be vitally important. It's much easier and much more accurate to measure food by weight. All of the recipes I develop are made using a food scale and then translated into American standard measurements using cups and spoons.

CHEESECLOTH

—

Cheesecloth is something that I always like to have on hand. It can be used in place of a nut milk bag or a strainer, or it could even be used in place of a tofu press when trying to remove liquids from a solid. I've wrapped plenty of vegan meats with cheesecloth to keep textures firmer while cooking but also allow liquid to cook off.

HIGH-POWERED BLENDER

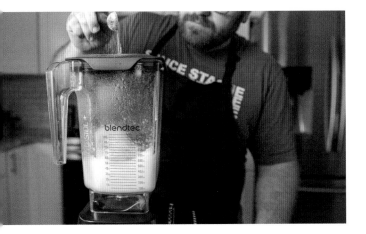

One of my most used tools by far is my blender. I would strongly recommend that anyone who has a standard blender upgrade to a more powerful blender. A high-powered blender allows you to create finer blends to make better-consistency products, and it will also allow you to mix thicker and denser mixtures then a basic home blender. I use a Blendtec blender, and it's by far one of my favorite kitchen tools.

STEAMER POT
—

Steaming is a necessity when making plant-based meats. It's a form of slow cooking using wet heat. Water boils at around 212°F, so when steaming, that is the highest temperature your food will be cooked at. It's the preferred method to cook loads of veggies, but also how I like to cook seitan. Owning a steamer pot will change the way you cook at home. There are a ton of varieties of steamer pots, from insert bamboo steamers that go on top of pots or pans to whole pots that have steamers built in. Any one of these products will work; as long as you

can put a lid on your pan to retain the steam, you are good to go!

POTS, PANS, AND IRON SKILLETS
—

You'll need pots, pans, and skillets to get through a cooking book. Why do people add this part to their books? You'll also need forks, spoons, and knives to eat. Oh, and whisks, cups, ladles, spatulas... You need cooking supplies to cook, is where I'm going. Wait...

SPATULAS
—

Get the ones that are soft silicone. Those are my favorite.

EXPERIMENT

I say this a lot in this book. It's the key to perfecting plant-based meats. Every time I try something new, I find out something else that I wouldn't have thought of. You might be trying to make some great vegan bacon, but then notice that the texture is really firm or really fatty and that might make a better steak, or a thinly sliced meat replacement, or maybe dry it to make a really great jerky.

I enjoy reading. I love seeing what other plant-based chefs do, seeing what they create. Maybe their already awesome recipe can be a jumping point for you to create your own incredible recipe. I hope that's what my book does for you. I hope you can use my recipes, swap the flavors, textures, and binders, and create something new for you!

I always try to really dial in textures first. That is the hardest in a lot of recipes. If you can get something close to the texture, then the taste isn't far away.

Take a look at nutrition labels, look at how much protein something has, how much fat, how much fiber. You can use these percentages to figure out your next plant-based meat recipe. That ground beef that's 80/20 tells you right away that, when you make a veggie burger, you should shoot for adding 20 percent fat by weight to your recipe.

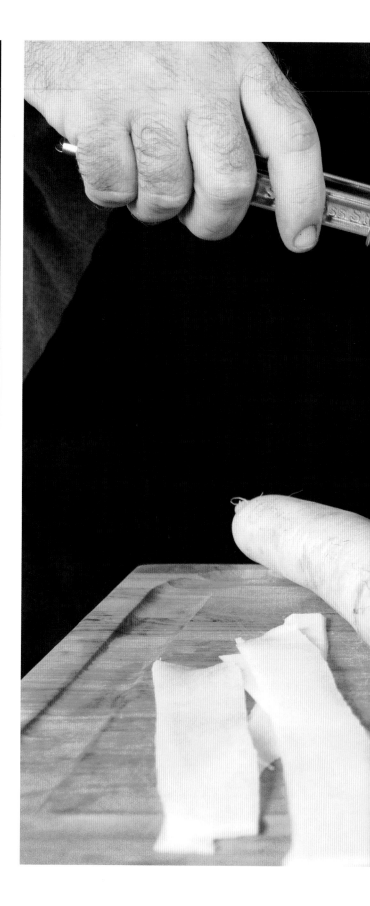

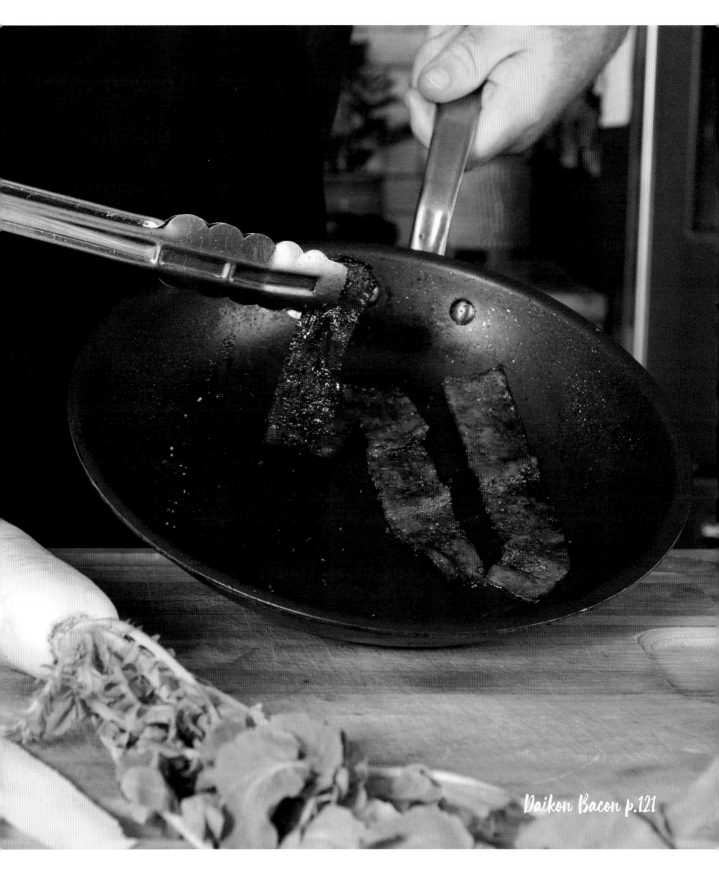

Daikon Bacon p.121

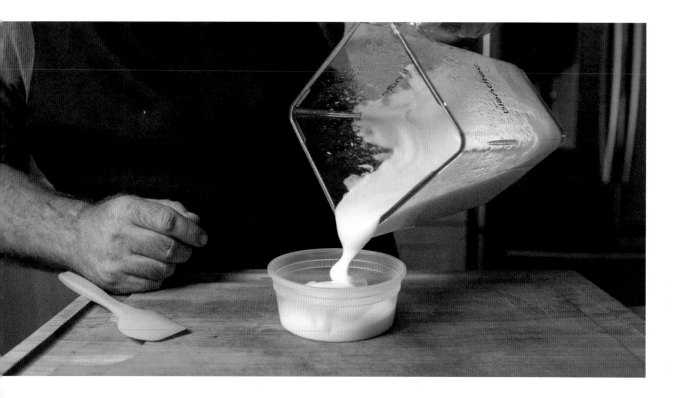

Making Meat Fat

The fat marbling in any meat is one of the most important things to recreate to get texture, sizzle, and mouthfeel out of your plant-based meats. This is my basic version of the meat fat. I always make it ahead of time because you can freeze the fat and have it ready to be shredded into almost any plant-based meat recipe. This will work to flavor beef, pork, or chicken recipes.

Divide this recipe into four separate freezable containers. Each container will have enough fat for one pound of plant-based meat.

To experiment with this, I have also added a carrageenan or agar agar to the mix to create a firmer marbling for steaks. Beyond Burger uses cocoa butter in their marbling mixture, which can also be used here as well. You can add flavors and salts. Vegan chicken stock added to the fat for a chicken recipe would also be a great experimental addition.

This makes enough "fat" for four pounds of plant-based meat. I divide this recipe into four plastic containers, then freeze. This animal-fat simulator will work in every recipe that calls for fat. I have created a lot of my recipes simply by experimenting with known methods of making plant-based meat and adding layers or chunks of simulated meat fat. The fat can create layers or pockets in seitan, TVP, or layered vegetables and mushrooms. The gum and methylcellulose will help bind the layers together but, when experimenting, make sure your texture has its own binder strong enough to bond the layers on its own.

INGREDIENTS

¾ CUP WATER

1 TEASPOON METHYLCELLULOSE

½ TEASPOON XANTHAN GUM

1½ CUPS REFINED COCONUT OIL

DIRECTIONS

- Add water to blender and start on slow speed with lid removed.
- Add methylcellulose and xanthan gum to blender and allow to gel.
- Keep blender spinning on slow speed and *very* slowly drip in coconut oil.
- Once you see coconut oil combining with the water/gel mixture, start to slowly transition from drip to a very slow stream in the coconut oil, and stream until all coconut oil has been added.
- This should now be an almost mayo-like consistency.
- Separate into 4 small freezer-safe containers and freeze until solid.
- Each fat puck is the equivalent fat for 1 pound of ground meat.

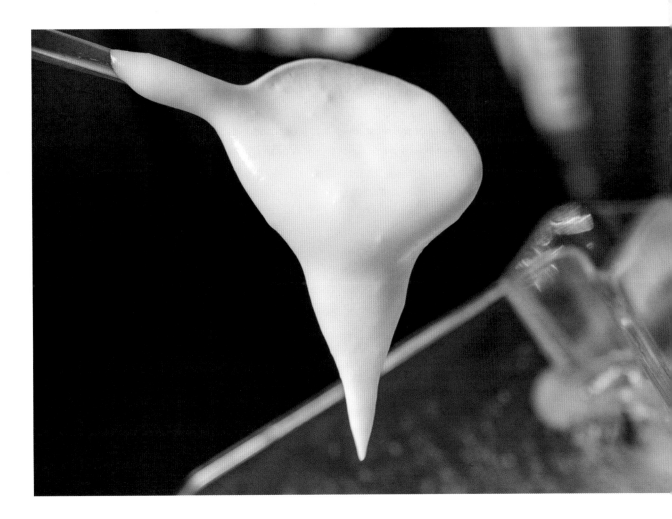

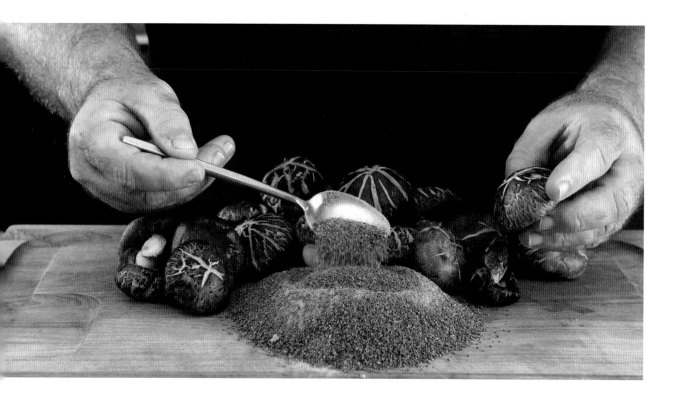

Making Pure Umami Mushroom Powder

I use mushroom powder in most of my recipes. It's something that can be substituted with a small amount of MSG. This is my version of mushroom powder or mushroom seasoning mix. It will really give you a nice savory punch in a small dose.

I do recommend picking up mushroom seasoning from your local Asian market or at amazon.com/shop/saucestache.

But for those of you who want to make it from scratch, here is my best attempt at it!

Make it, then let me know what you think on social media using #saucestache.

I use mushroom seasoning powder in most of my recipes. Mushroom seasoning is a great addition to most recipes, but in vegan meat, it really adds that savory umami boost that a lot of vegan meat recipes really need. I strongly recommend finding mushroom seasoning powder online or at your local Asian market. This homemade version will work if mushroom seasoning is too difficult to find in your area.

INGREDIENTS

2 POUNDS FRESH SHIITAKE
    MUSHROOMS

2 POUNDS DRIED SHIITAKE
    MUSHROOMS

SALT

ABOUT 20 CUPS FILTERED WATER

3 TABLESPOONS SALT

DIRECTIONS

- Clean the fresh mushrooms with a brush and remove any damaged stems.
- Place the mushrooms in a large Dutch oven or stock pot, cover with filtered water, and add half the salt. Cover with lid and bring to a boil. Once at a boil, lower heat to keep at a simmer. Simmer for 2 hours, checking throughout to make sure more water isn't needed.
- After 2 hours, we are going to save the liquid mushroom broth and then cover the mushrooms again with water and the other half of the salt. Repeat the previous step.
- Once the mushrooms are done boiling, remove them and place in a clean dry cotton cloth or cheesecloth, then squeeze as much liquid out of the mushrooms as possible into the mushroom broth.
- Combine both broths and simmer on medium heat until the mushroom broth liquid is reduced by three-quarters.
- Now, using the dried mushrooms, put them in a blender and blend until you have a fine mushroom powder.
- Combine the mushroom powder with the reduced broth and mix well.
- On a parchment-paper-lined baking sheet, spread out the mixture very thin.
- Place in an oven on lowest setting to dehydrate. Depending on your location, the time of year, and oven temp, this process can take 6–8 hours. You want this to be fully dehydrated and very dry.
- Once the mushrooms are fully dehydrated, put back in blender to blend into a fine powder.
- This is where you can customize your taste. I want this mixture to be salty. I will add salt to the powder until I get a nice punchy, salty, savory flavor. If you want a less salty flavor, you can stop now.

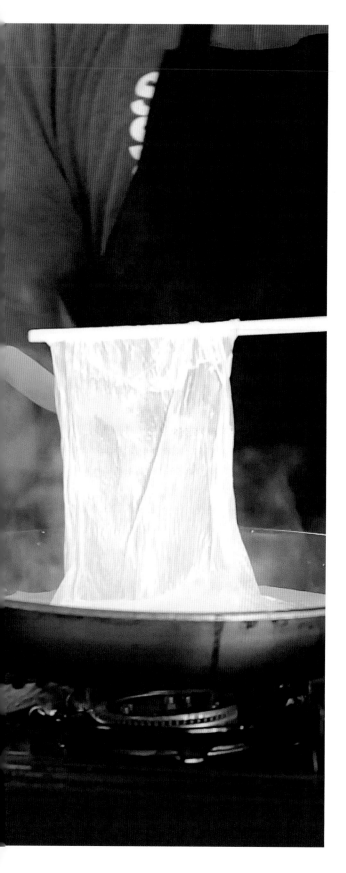

Making Soy Skin

I use soy skin quite a bit. It goes by the names soy skin, tofu skin, yuba, and I'm sure a few others. You can buy dried or fresh soy skin at just about any Asian market, and you can find it dried online fairly easily. Sometimes you need to make it in a pinch, or freshly made soy skin is sometimes just easier to work with.

Either way, it's fairly simple and you only need one ingredient, soy milk, or soybeans if you want to make it from scratch...scratch. Once you have it made, it might take a little practice to handle. It's thin, and sticky, and it sticks to itself fairly easily, but once you've got it, it's worth it as the best fake meat skin I know. Make it, experiment with it. Try it as a textured product or wrap up some veggies with it to make them more realistic meat replacements.

INGREDIENTS

½ GALLON SOY MILK

OR

1 CUP DRIED SOYBEANS SOAKED
    OVERNIGHT IN WATER

3 CUPS WATER

DIRECTIONS

- If you are going to make this from the bean, then you need to make the milk first.
- Blend your 1 cup of soaked beans with the 3 cups water until you have a soy cream.
- Pour the mixture through a strainer, then through a nut milk bag, or one of those Thai tea bags I was talking about earlier.
- You now have soy milk.
- To make your soy skin, fill a nonstick skillet to the top with soy milk and bring your heat to a low/medium-low heat. You will want to heat the milk slowly so it doesn't burn.
- Once the mixture starts to steam and slightly simmer, you should see a film forming at the top. The first skin takes the longest to form. As soon as you see this skin starting to form, bump up the heat just a touch.
- The skin will start to get slightly thicker and form over the entire surface of the soy milk in the pan and stick to the edges of the pan. You might even see a large bubble starting to form.
- Quickly run a spatula around the edges of the pan to release the skin from the pan, then use a chopstick or other long thin utensil to lift the skin off the top of the pan.
- You can hang these around the edge of a large bowl, or over the side of a counter, to drip and slightly dry, or you can immediately wrap them around your "meat" to make a skin.

BEEF

Plant-based burgers, steaks, deli meats, and even plant-based ground meats can be made in so many different ways. Using gluten, plant proteins, textured products, vegetables, and mushrooms the possibilities are endless.

Most of the recipes in the beef section can be manipulated and tweaked to your liking. You can make them more savory using more yeasts or flavor extracts, and the proteins are interchangeable.

I am still always experimenting with making a better plant-based beef. Texture is just as important as taste and smell, and appearance wrap it into a nice package. The recipes ahead are some of my favorite attempts at making plant-based beef better.

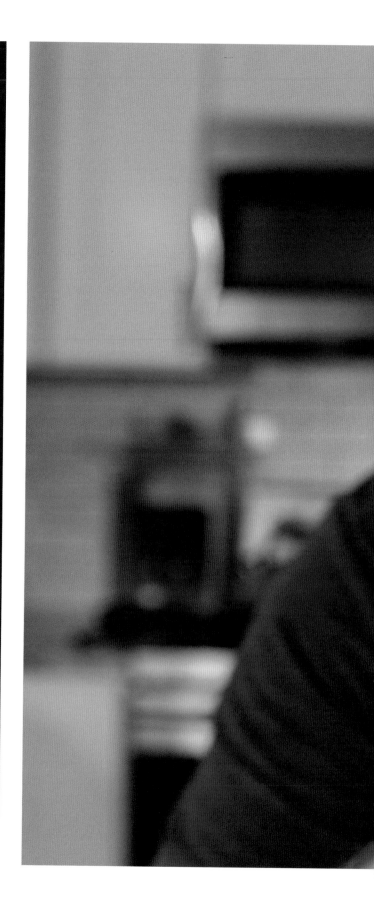

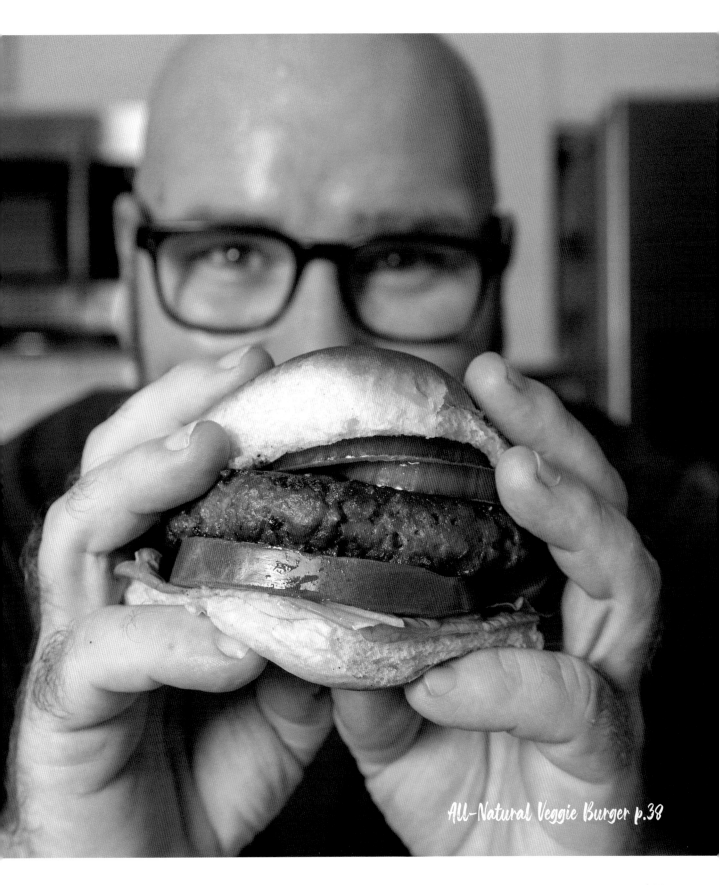

All-Natural Veggie Burger p.38

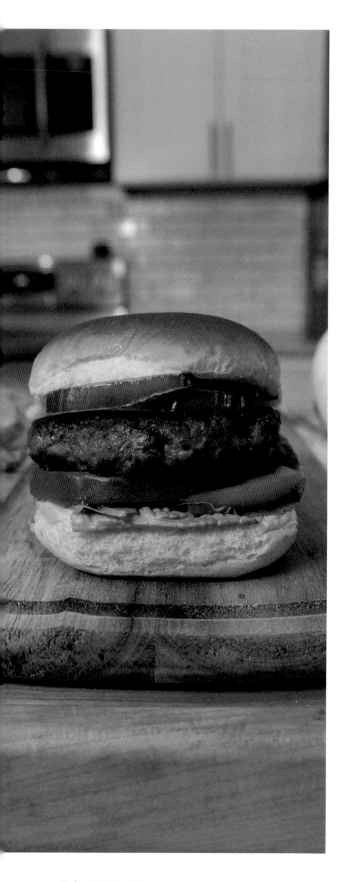

All-Natural Veggie Burger

This first recipe was inspired by a video I saw, based on a burger created by Chef David of Planta. It is a combination of legumes, oats, and seasonings to create an incredibly meaty veggie burger that is all veg! Mostly simple ingredients, and incredibly easy to make on the fly.

This one has a bunch of options, but you can always try making these substitutions:

- 3 portobellos for a half pound of any mushroom; try shiitake for extra-meaty taste
- 1½ tablespoons nutritional yeast for 1 tablespoon Marmite
- Tapioca starch for potato starch
- 1 tablespoon soy sauce for 1 tablespoon liquid aminos

This burger is best made thin, topped with your favorite vegan cheese slice and your favorite burger toppings! Whip up some of my favorite spicy mayo burger topping.

- 2 tablespoons vegan mayo
- 1 teaspoon tabasco chipotle sauce
- ½ teaspoons smoked paprika
- 1 teaspoon finely minced onions
- Mix everything together in a bowl

INGREDIENTS

3 LARGE PORTOBELLO MUSHROOMS
(OR MUSHROOMS OF CHOICE)

¼ YELLOW ONION

1 CAN OF BLACK BEANS (DRAINED
AND RINSED)

3 TABLESPOONS CANNED
CHICKPEAS

3 TABLESPOONS CHICKPEA WATER
(AQUAFABA)

1 TABLESPOON BEET JUICE FROM
CAN OF BEETS

1–2 TABLESPOONS OF CHOPPED
BEET FROM CAN

½ TEASPOON GARLIC POWDER

1 TEASPOON LIQUID SMOKE

1 TEASPOON BLACKSTRAP
MOLASSES

1 TABLESPOON SOY SAUCE

3 TABLESPOONS LENTILS FROM CAN
(WASHED AND RINSED)

BONUS ½ TEASPOON MUSHROOM
EXTRACT POWDER (FOR ADDED
UMAMI)

¾ CUP OATS

1½ TABLESPOON NUTRITIONAL
YEAST

2 TABLESPOONS TAPIOCA STARCH
(TAPIOCA FLOUR)

DIRECTIONS

- Coarsely chop mushrooms and onion.
- Toss into frying pan with oil over medium heat and give a slight toss.
- Stir mushrooms and onions to make sure they are coated in oil.
- Add the beans, chickpeas, beets, and liquid into a food processor or blender and pulse together.
- Be careful not to over-pulse. You want the mixture to have a rough texture, not smooth.
- Now add your garlic powder, liquid smoke, molasses, and soy sauce into the food processor or blender and quickly pulse. Add your lentils, and mushroom extract if you have it, and briefly pulse.
- Remove mixture from food processor and add to a medium bowl. Now add oats, nutritional yeast, and tapioca starch. Mix together well by hand.
- Heat a skillet over medium to low heat with a small amount of cooking oil (I use olive oil).
- Make patties **thin**. You want these burgers to be roughly the same thickness as a fast-food burger.
- TIP: Wet your hands with cold water to form patties!
- Season with a little salt and pepper to taste.
- Drop burger patties in skillet with a tablespoon of olive oil. Let cook 3–4 minutes each side. Cook each side only once!

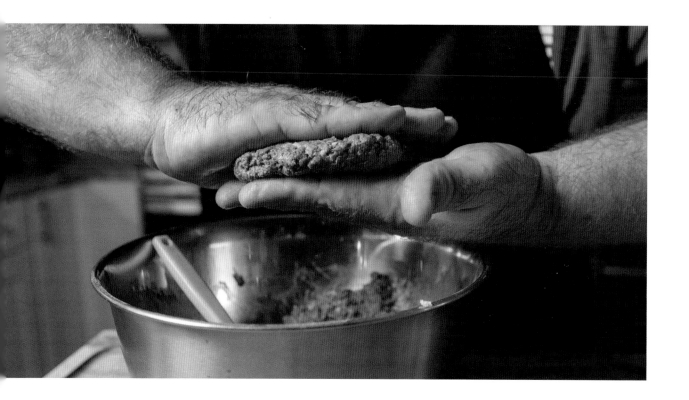

Textured Protein Burger

I first messed with textured vegetable protein when making a vegan chili. When I started seeing more meat-like burgers come to market, I noticed their heavy use of textured protein, and that is when I attempted to make a copy of one of those vegan burgers that seemed impossible to make. This is that recipe.

One of my favorite things about this recipe is that it is a base for any ground beef recipe *and* the base of this recipe can be swapped around to make ground-almost-anything. The parts that need to stick around are the TVP, protein, methylcellulose, and fat. Using those four ingredients with these measurements and swapping out the flavors can really change what you end up with. Make it savory, a little sweet, and a little smoky, and you have a great ground pork base. Remove the savory flavors

and throw in a vegan chicken broth instead of water, and you end up with a super simple ground chicken.

Experiment away with this one because the possibilities are endless.

You can swap anything here!
- 4 tablespoons potato protein for pea protein (or any powdered protein mix you like)
- ½ teaspoon mushroom extract powder for ¼ teaspoon MSG
- ½ teaspoon beetroot powder + 1 cup water for 1 cup beet juice
- 3 tablespoons nutritional yeast for 2 tablespoons Marmite
- 1 teaspoon soy sauce for 1 teaspoon liquid aminos

I love this burger topped all the way! A little vegan cheese, lettuce, tomato, onion, fried garlic, and some vegan mayo...but if you want to take it over the top:

- 1 small can mushrooms
- 1 teaspoon Marmite
- 1 tablespoon vegan butter

Mix mushrooms and Marmite together. Heat vegan butter in a skillet over medium heat and toss mushrooms until cooked through.

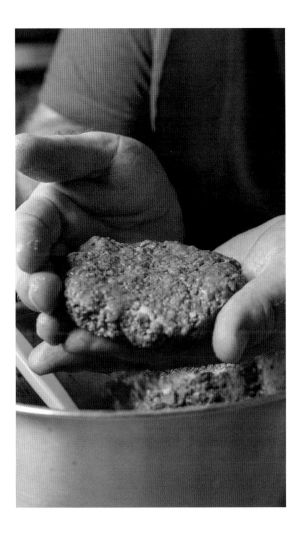

INGREDIENTS

1 CUP TVP

4 TABLESPOONS POTATO PROTEIN

1 TABLESPOON METHYLCELLULOSE, HIGH-VISCOSITY

½ TEASPOON MUSHROOM EXTRACT POWDER (OR ANY MUSHROOM POWDER)

½ TEASPOON ONION POWDER

½ TEASPOON GARLIC POWDER

1 TEASPOON BEETROOT POWDER

3 TABLESPOONS NUTRITIONAL YEAST

1 CUP WATER

½ TEASPOON LIQUID SMOKE

½ TEASPOON BLACKSTRAP MOLASSES

1 TEASPOON SOY SAUCE

½ TEASPOON WHITE VINEGAR

1 FROZEN FAT SIMULATOR (SEE BURGER FAT RECIPE ON PAGE 30)

DIRECTIONS

- Mix dry ingredients together really well in a large bowl.
- Mix wet ingredients together in separate bowl or cup.
- Mix dry and wet ingredients well.
- Allow mixture to sit covered for at least 30 minutes. This allows the TVP and methylcellulose to hydrate. Without this hydrating time, the TVP texture won't be correct, and the methylcellulose won't work when cooking!
- Shred frozen fat, using a large grater, into burger and mix well.
- Form burger patty. These burgers can be thick or thin and can be cooked in a skillet or on a grill!
- I cook in a skillet with a touch of oil over medium heat for 4–6 minutes a side, flipping only once!

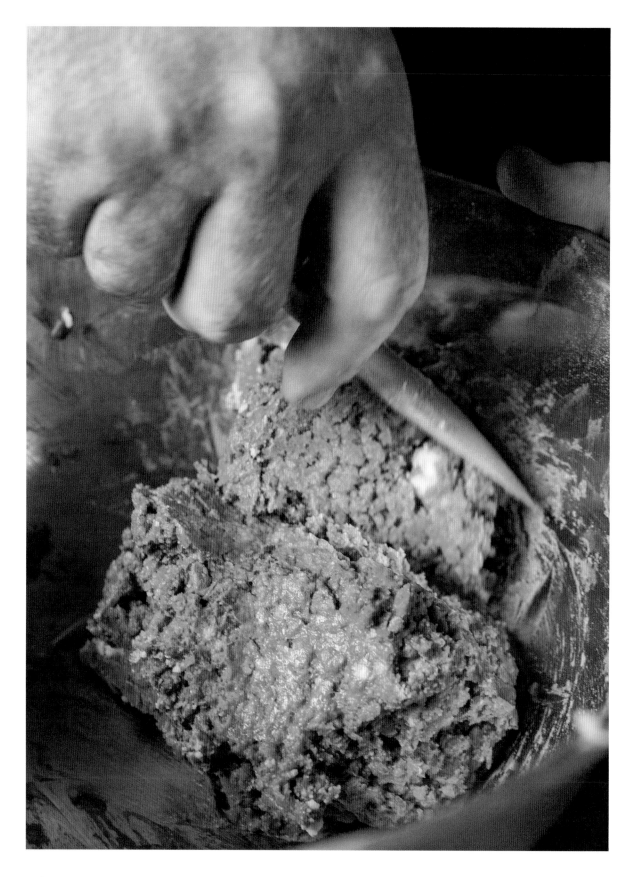

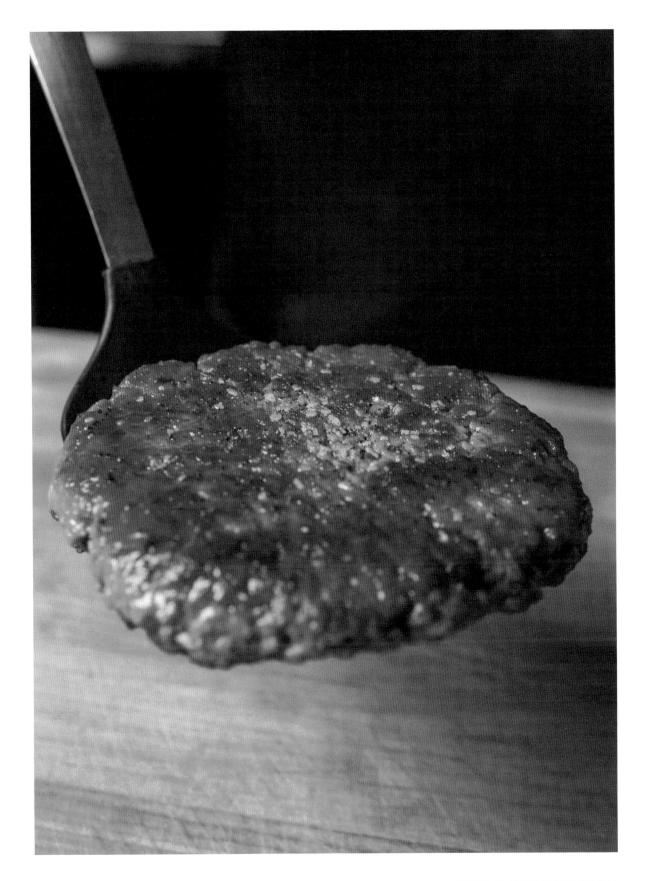

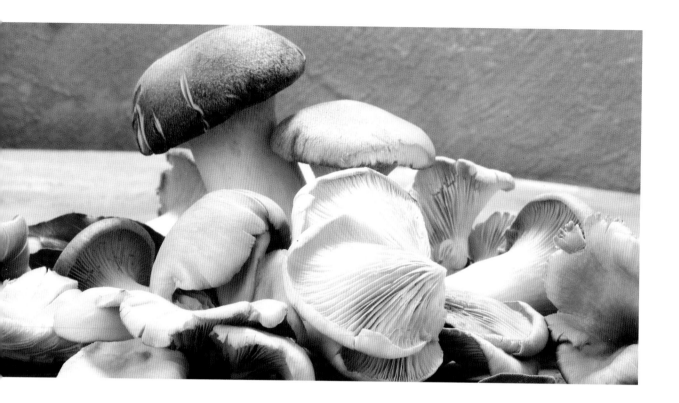

Mushroom Burger

I love mushrooms and all their incredible flavors and textures! They are irreplaceable in the plant-based meat world. Using mushrooms whole in plant-based meats is common but it's also fun to grind them up, or at least give them a good rough chopping to make an incredible textured mushroom burger.

This is a perfect example of using a different texture source with similar flavor ingredients to come up with a fantastic burger.

You can also try swapping out two portobello mushrooms chopped for 6 oz of baby bellas, or 6 oz of shiitake mushrooms OR any mushroom.

- 1 teaspoon soy sauce for 1 teaspoon liquid aminos
- Try adding a tablespoon of Marmite to make it even meatier.

Make sure to top this burger with a slice of your favorite vegan cheese! I *love* to top these burgers with a slab of A.1. sauce!

INGREDIENTS

2 PORTOBELLO MUSHROOMS
    CHOPPED

¼ MEDIUM YELLOW ONION CHOPPED

1 TEASPOON BLACKSTRAP
    MOLASSES

1 TEASPOON LIQUID SMOKE

2 PINCHES OF SALT

1 TEASPOON SOY SAUCE

1 TEASPOON GARLIC POWDER

½ CUP OATS

⅓ CUP EGG REPLACER (SEE EGG
    REPLACERS FOR CHOICES)

¼ CUP VITAL WHEAT GLUTEN

DIRECTIONS

- Cook onions over medium heat in nonstick skillet with a drop of olive oil and a pinch of salt. Toss to cover. Allow onions to cook until translucent.
- Once the onions are cooked, add all of the ingredients except vital wheat gluten in a large bowl and mix them together.
- Once mixed, add vital wheat gluten. Mix together, then knead by hand to form gluten bond. The more you knead the denser the texture will be. You will feel the texture change from soft and squishy to a denser patty.
- Allow mixture to sit for 15 minutes, then form thin fast-food-style burgers by hand.
- Season both sides with salt and pepper to taste.
- These burgers will do well on the grill or skillet, cooking each side for 4–5 minutes over a medium heat.

Vegan Wagyu Steak—Marbled Seitan

I have always been chasing the perfect steak replacement, along with just about every commercial plant-based meat maker. So far no one has nailed it...except I think this is pretty dang close. It's marbled and steaky. You can add more marbling or less. This can be cooked in a skillet, as I do, or thrown on a grill for that flame taste.

All of these can be swapped out and interchanged! Experiment!

- ¼ cup chickpea flour for ¼ cup canned chickpeas
- 2 tablespoons Marmite for 2½ tablespoons nutritional yeast
- 1 tablespoon mushroom extract powder for 1 tsp MSG
- ½ tablespoon kappa carrageenan for 1 tablespoon agar agar
- 2 tablespoons soy sauce for 2 tablespoons liquid aminos
- 1 teaspoon beetroot powder + 1 cup water for 1 cup beet juice

Pair this with a quick garlic mashed potato.

- 3 russet potatoes
- 1 cup plant-based milk (I have been loving pea protein milk)
- 6 cloves crushed garlic
- 2 tablespoons nutritional yeast
- 2 tablespoons vegan butter
- Salt and pepper to taste

Peel and cube potatoes, then boil in a large saucepan filled with salted water. Cook until potatoes are very soft and can be pressed with a fork.

Drain potatoes and return to saucepan. Add plant milk, crushed garlic, nutritional yeast, and vegan butter, then mash with potato masher.

Salt and pepper to taste.

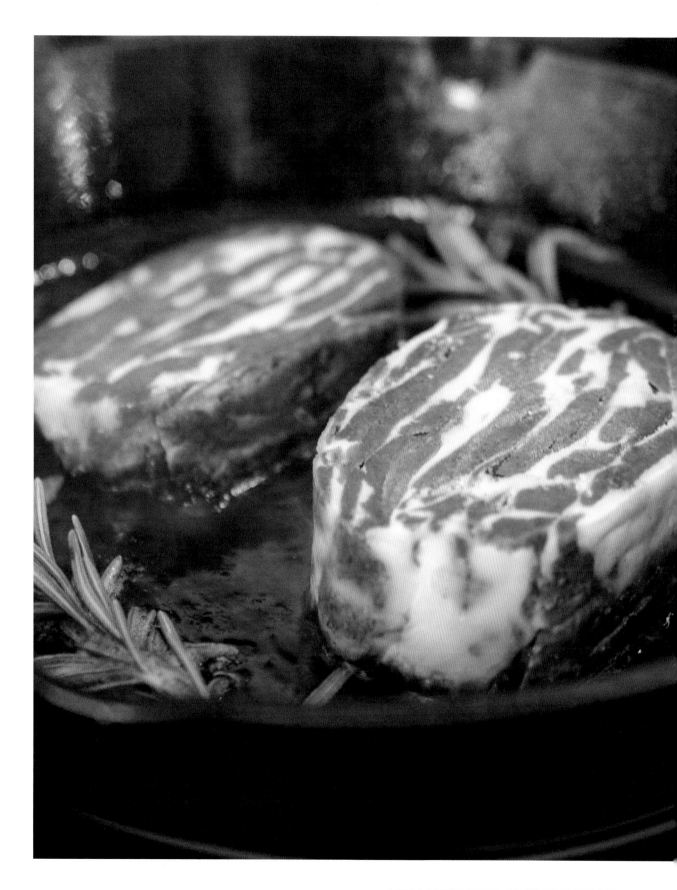

INGREDIENTS

MEAT

2 CUPS VITAL WHEAT GLUTEN

¼ CUP CHICKPEA FLOUR

2 TABLESPOONS OIL (I USED OLIVE
   OIL)

2 TABLESPOONS MARMITE (OR
   NUTRITIONAL YEAST)

2 TABLESPOONS SOY SAUCE

1 TABLESPOON MUSHROOM
   EXTRACT POWDER

1 TABLESPOON VINEGAR

1 TEASPOON LIQUID SMOKE

1 TABLESPOON BLACKSTRAP
   MOLASSES

½ CUP WATER

FAT

¾ CUP WATER

1 TEASPOON METHYLCELLULOSE

1 CUP REFINED COCONUT OIL

½ TABLESPOON KAPPA
   CARRAGEENAN

BROTH

1 TEASPOON BEETROOT POWDER

1 TEASPOON COCOA POWDER

1 CUP WATER

PINCH OF SALT

DIRECTIONS

- Add all of the meat ingredients to the jar of a high-powered blender or to a food processor and pulse to combine. You should end up with a ground beef consistency.
- Pour ground mixture onto a clean work surface and knead until everything is combined. This should be a very firm dough ball. Cover and let rest while completing the next steps.
- Now we are going to make the fat, very similar to how we make our fat pucks for burger recipes. Add water to the jar of a blender and start blender on lowest speed.
- Slowly add methylcellulose until fully combined.
- While blender is still spinning on low, start dripping in coconut oil, then increase drip to a slow drizzle. If you pour oil too quickly, it will not combine.
- Keep the blender moving on a slow speed and add the kappa carrageenan. Blend for a moment to mix. Now you can stop the blender and you should have a mayo-like consistency.
- Now we are going to build our steaks. Using a large sheet of parchment paper, place a dollop of your fat mixture and spread flat in the middle of the parchment paper.
- Take your rested meat dough ball and slice very thin slices of meat, similar to deli meat slices. Then cut those slices into thin noodle-like strips.
- Place the strips tightly together, all in the same direction, on the fat. Continue laying the strips of meat on the fat until you have a meat layer around the size of your hand.
- Place another dollop of fat on top of your meat layer and continue this layering until you are out of meat.
- Once you are out of meat, your last layer should be a fat layer that covers your entire meat loaf.
- Tightly wrap the loaf, then wrap in a layer of foil or plastic wrap.
- Bring a large pot of water to a boil and place wrapped steak loaf in water. Boil for 45 minutes.
- Remove from boiling water and place in freezer to cool down and set the carrageenan. This could take around an hour.
- Make your broth by combining all broth ingredients and mix well. Remove firm steak loaf from freezer, unwrap, and trim into 2 large

steaks or 4 small steaks. Always cut the steaks against the grain. You want the grain to be vertical in your steak.

- Place trimmed steaks into broth and refrigerate 6 hours, or overnight is best.
- Cook steaks on grill or in a hot skillet with some oil.

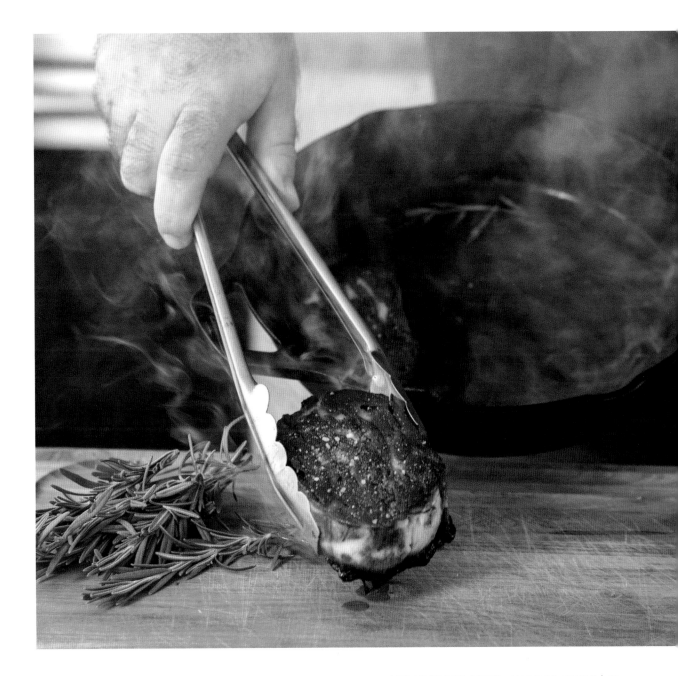

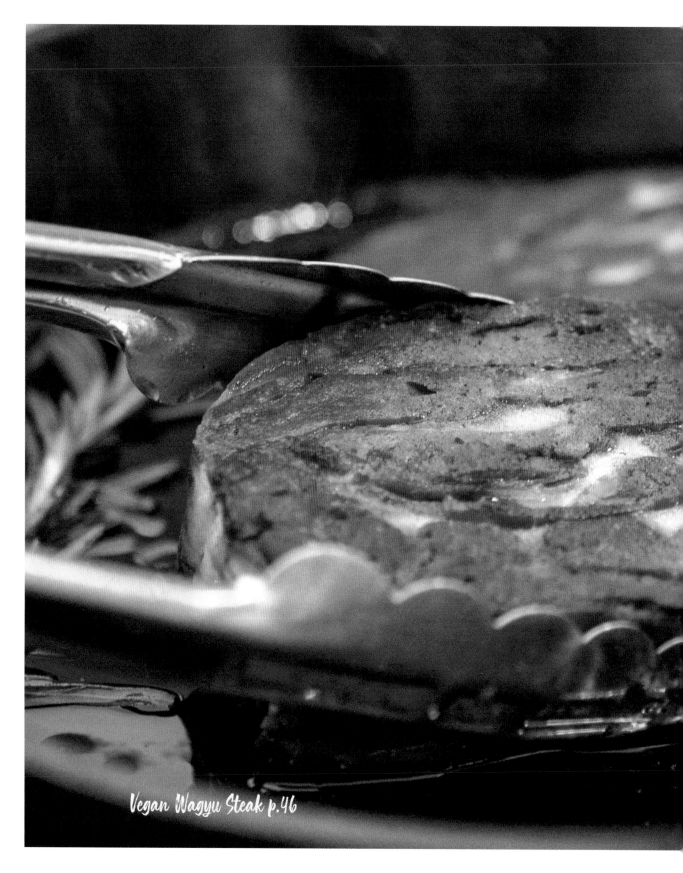

Vegan Wagyu Steak p.46

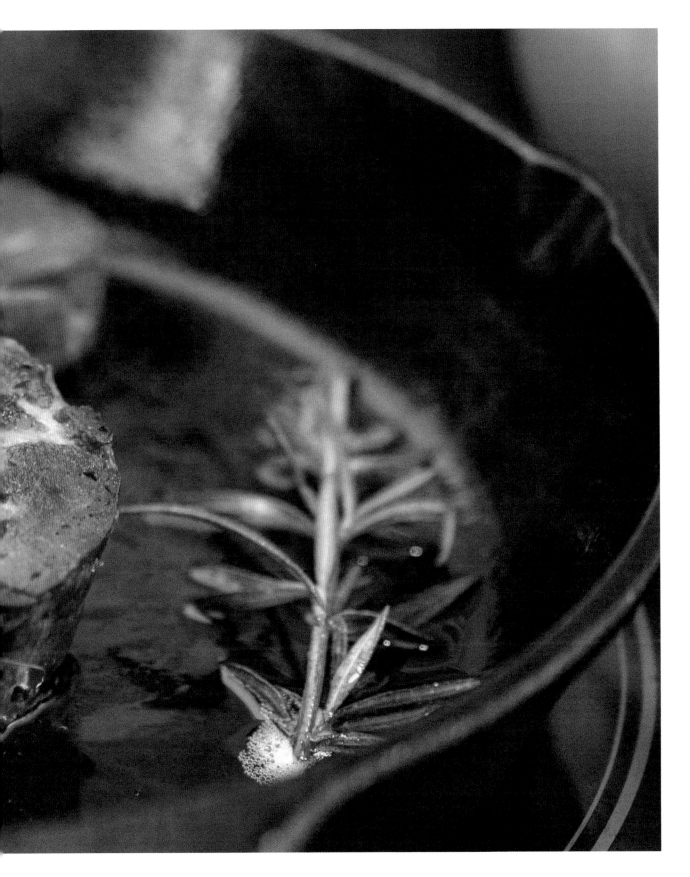

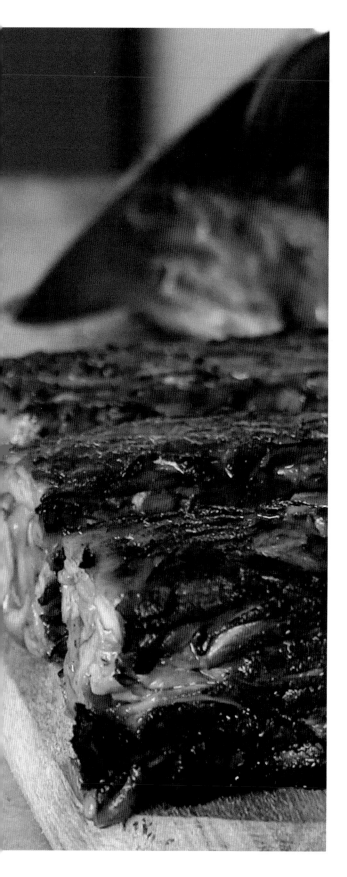

Textured Mushroom Steak

This next steak I actually dreamt about. In my mind, I put a steak together similar to how a croissant is made. I hoped that layering fat and binder between mushrooms would create a steak-like texture that broke when you chewed it, but also had the constancy of a mushroom. This is one of the more unique recipes in the book, as it is not so much as a faux meat or meat replacement as its very own unique new thing.

Swap out the mushrooms for any other mushroom.

You will absolutely love this steak with some sautéed mushroom, onions, and garlic mixed with a pinch of Marmite and liquid smoke.

INGREDIENTS

2 POUNDS OF KING OYSTER
    MUSHROOMS

2 TABLESPOONS OLIVE OIL

2 TABLESPOONS NUTRITIONAL
    YEAST

1 TSP MARMITE

1 TSP BLACKSTRAP MOLASSES

2 TABLESPOONS SOY SAUCE

1 TABLESPOON RICE VINEGAR

1 TABLESPOON MUSHROOM
    EXTRACT POWDER

2 TEASPOONS BEETROOT POWDER

1 TABLESPOON VINEGAR

1 TEASPOON LIQUID SMOKE

1 TEASPOON BEEF-FLAVORED
    BROTH MIX

2 TABLESPOONS PEA PROTEIN
    POWDER

1 TABLESPOON METHYLCELLULOSE

1 TABLESPOON KAPPA
    CARRAGEENAN

½ CUP WATER

1 SEPARATE CUP WATER FOR
    FLAVOR

DIRECTIONS

- Clean and peel your mushrooms. I peel the mushrooms, but I have shredded the mushrooms using the method I saw from Derek Sarno, taking 2 forks and pulling the mushrooms into fine shreds. Set aside in large bowl.
- Make your binder and color by adding water to a blender and starting your blender on a slow speed, then slowly adding methylcellulose followed by kappa carrageenan. Once this forms into a thick "whipped cream" consistency, add broth mix and beetroot powder.
- Toss the mushrooms with pea protein and nutritional yeast, then mix with vinegar and soy sauce.
- Make flavor broth with 1 cup water, Marmite, molasses, and liquid smoke. Mix well, then mix with mushrooms. Allow to soak for 30 minutes.
- Using a large sheet of parchment paper, place about 2 tablespoons worth of your pink binder mix on the parchment paper and spread out into a roughly 8 x 5-inch rectangle (about the size of a small loaf of bread). Create one layer of mushroom by laying mushrooms in a horizontal even row.
- Now create layers, almost like a lasagna! Mushroom, binder, mushroom, binder, until you've used up all your mushrooms.
- Wrap your mushroom steak tightly in the parchment paper, then double-wrap in foil, pressing tight and wrapping very firm.
- Place in a shallow pan or baking sheet and bake at 350°F until internal temp reaches 160°F (about an hour).
- Remove from the oven and place a heavy pan or cast-iron skillet on top of the cooked mushrooms to press. Once cooled to room temp, remove skillet and place mushrooms in the refrigerator overnight.
- Unwrap from parchment paper and cut your steaks (I was able to get 4 steaks), then add salt and pepper to taste. You can sear these on a grill or in a nicely oiled skillet.

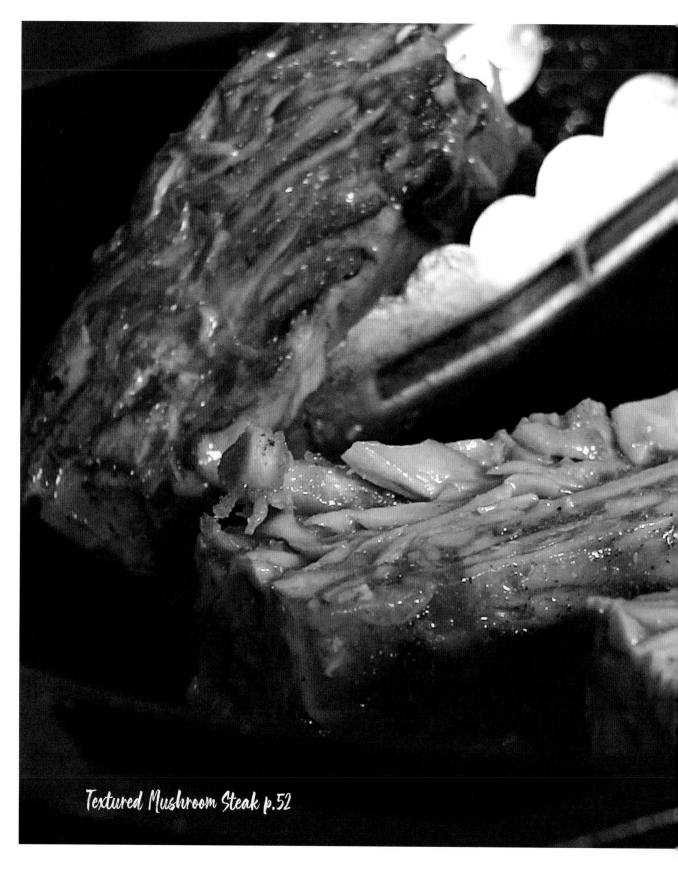

Textured Mushroom Steak p.52

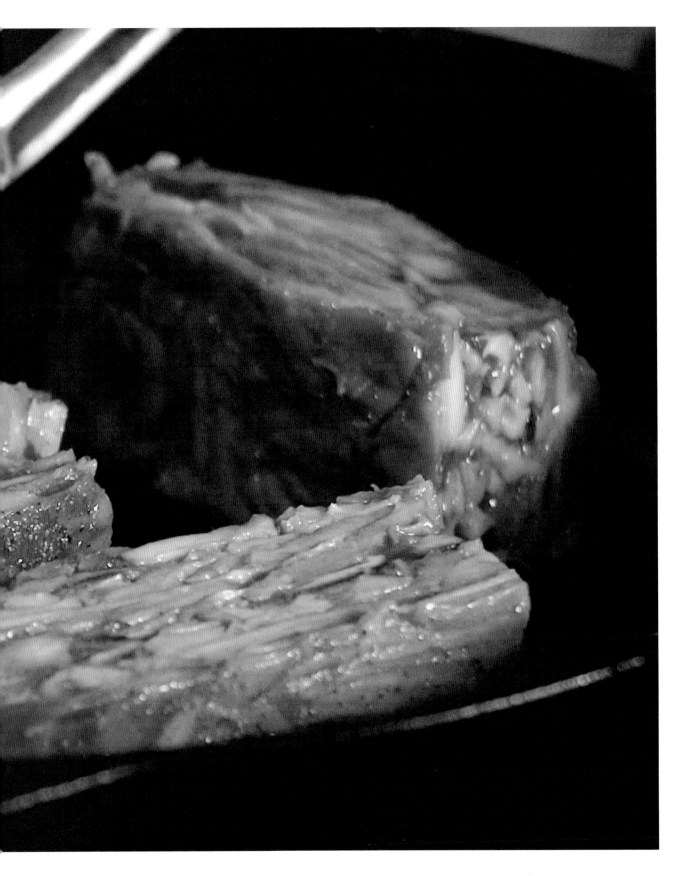

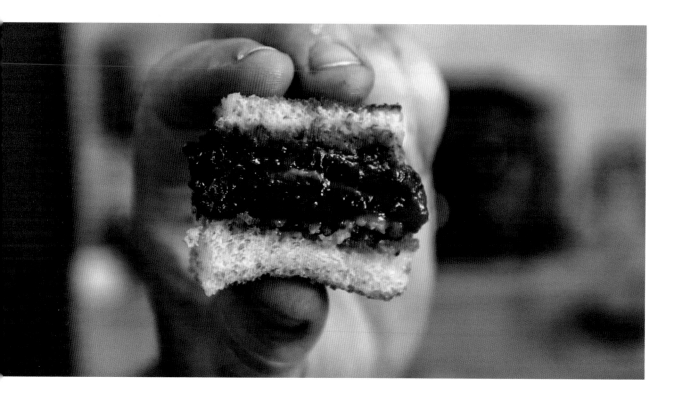

Watermelon Katsu Steak

After Ducks Eatery in New York premiered the watermelon steak, my interest was piqued in using watermelon as a meat replacement. I tried my hand at making watermelon ham (recipe further in the book) and I knew after that trial that I would have to take this watermelon experiment a heck of a lot further.

Watermelon as a vegan meat is an odd one for sure, and fun to play around with. Don't expect a perfect meat substitute but expect to have fun and end up with a really uniquely textured vegan meat similar to raw fish.

This is one to play around with for sure. I have used a similar recipe sliced thin to make a fun jerky-like bacon. I can't wait to see what you come up with.

Try adding Marmite or nutritional yeast for a meatier flavor, or you can really spice things up with a nice green sauce! Chimichurri! Add everything to a food processor or small blender and mix.

- 1 cup fresh parsley
- ½ cup fresh cilantro
- 2 tablespoons fresh oregano
- ½ cup olive oil
- 2 tablespoons red wine vinegar
- 1 teaspoon salt
- ½ teaspoon red pepper flakes
- 2 tablespoons lime juice
- 4 cloves garlic, chopped

INGREDIENTS

4 WATERMELON SLICES, 2 INCHES
   THICK

¼ CUP SOY SAUCE

¼ CUP WHITE VINEGAR

½ TABLESPOON LIQUID SMOKE

¼ TEASPOON PAPRIKA

1 TABLESPOON OLIVE OIL

1 TABLESPOON DARK BROWN
   SUGAR

SALT AND PEPPER TO TASTE

¼ CUP VEGAN BUTTER

SALT

BREADING

¼ CUP + 2 TABLESPOONS VEGAN
   EGG REPLACER

1 CUP FLOUR

1 CUP PANKO

½ TEASPOON SALT

VEGETABLE OIL FOR FRYING

DIRECTIONS

- Preheat oven to 350°F.
- Pat watermelon dry, then lightly salt and allow to sit on paper towel while you prepare the rest of the ingredients.
- Mix together soy sauce, vinegar, liquid smoke, paprika, olive oil, and brown sugar.
- Coat each slice of watermelon with mixture and place on baking sheet. Pour remaining mixture over the watermelon.
- Add a half-tablespoon of vegan butter on top of each slice of watermelon and bake for 1 hour and 45 minutes.
- Once baked, allow to cool enough to work with, and dip in flour, then egg mixture, then panko.
- Heat 1½ inches of oil in large pot until it reaches 350°F.
- Fry the watermelon pieces in small batches, constantly flipping until golden brown.
- Remove to rack or paper towel.

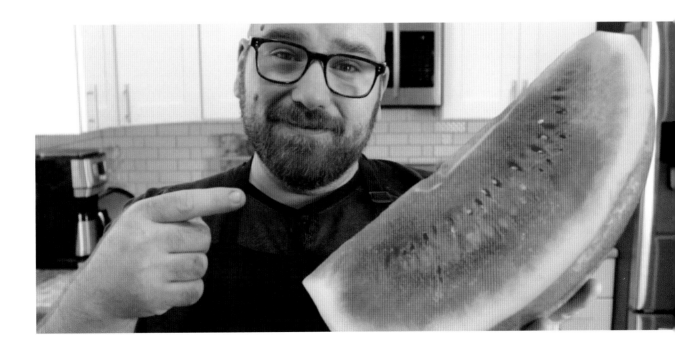

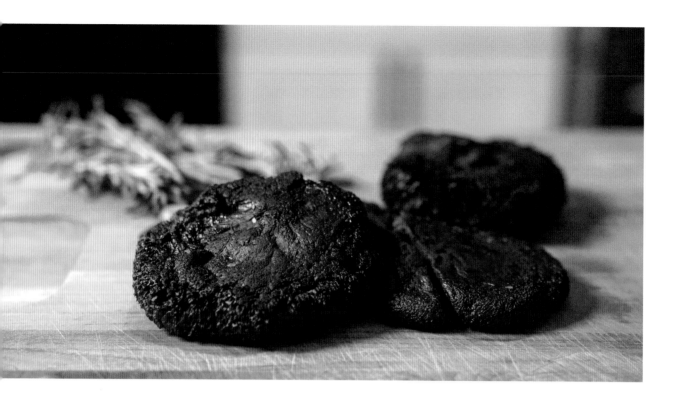

Lion's Mane Mushroom Steak

The last "steak" in the book is a steak made from mushrooms. Now my favorite part of this steak is how incredibly easy it is, how quick it goes together, and how great the texture is. We are still making a mushroom dish, but a mushroom dish that goes over the top on the steak taste! In this book we will explore fresh lion's mane mushrooms, but this recipe specifically calls for dried lion's mane.

This can be made a few ways. Try it how it is, but you can also slice the mushrooms really thin, then follow the same recipe and techniques to make a really unique deli meat. Just something else to experiment with and have fun. Try using the flavor broths from some of the bacons to turn this into a wild pork-chop-like mushroom!

Try changing 1 cup red wine for 1 tsp beetroot powder and 1 cup water or beet juice.

I have loved to pair this steak with Brussels sprouts. Sauté a pound of Brussels sprouts in a large cast-iron skillet over a high heat with around a tablespoon of olive oil. Give the skillet a shake every few moments until the sprouts are dark and caramelized. Add some salt, pepper, and a pinch of fresh finely chopped cilantro.

Remove from pan and drizzle with a squeeze of fresh lemon!

INGREDIENTS

4 DEHYDRATED LION'S MANE
    MUSHROOMS

3 CUPS WATER

½ CUP SOY SAUCE

1 CUP RED WINE

1 TEASPOON MARMITE

1 TABLESPOON MUSHROOM
    EXTRACT SEASONING

1 TABLESPOON VEGAN BEEF STOCK
    SEASONING

2 TABLESPOONS OLIVE OIL

1 TABLESPOON VEGAN BUTTER

1 SPRIG ROSEMARY

SALT AND PEPPER TO TASTE

DIRECTIONS

- In a saucepan, mix together water, soy sauce, wine, Marmite, mushroom extract, and vegan beef stock, and bring to a simmer. Once at a simmer, add mushrooms and cover. Cook for 30 minutes to rehydrate.
- Check water level, flipping halfway through, and add water if needed.
- Remove mushrooms from broth and press between two cutting boards to remove excess liquid. Press into small steak medallion shapes. You can use a tofu press or iron skillet for this as well. Press until mushroom holds its shape.
- Heat a large skillet over a medium high heat with olive oil and 1 or 2 sprigs rosemary. Salt and pepper both sides of your mushroom steak. Place in the skillet, then drop a small scoop of vegan butter on the mushroom. Once the butter has completely melted, flip over and press flat with your spatula. Spoon any remaining oil or butter over the mushroom steak and serve.

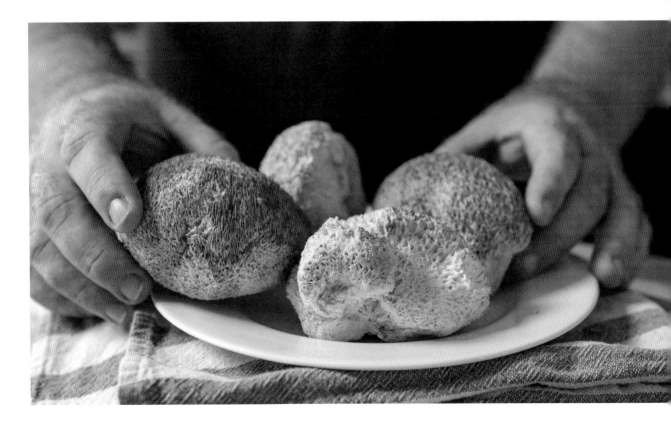

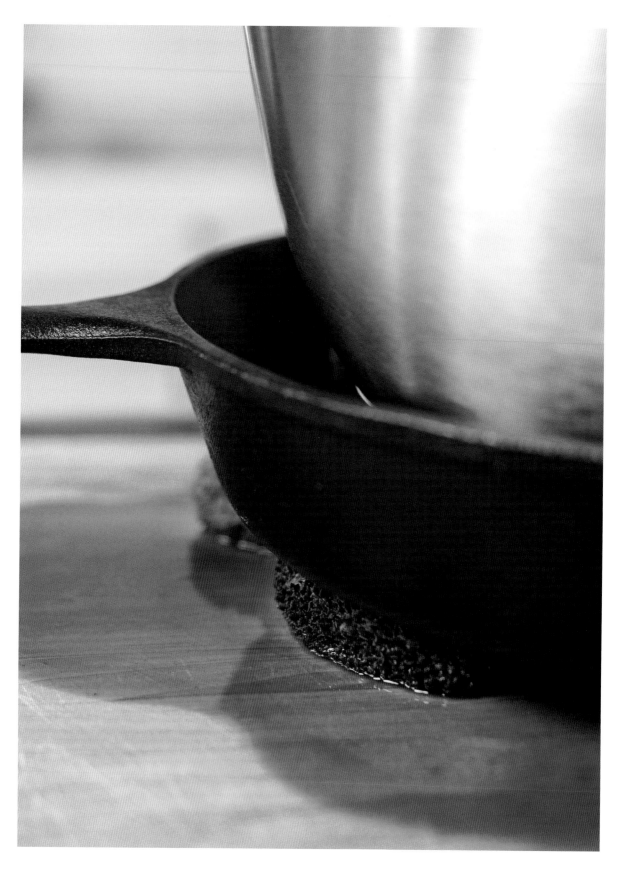

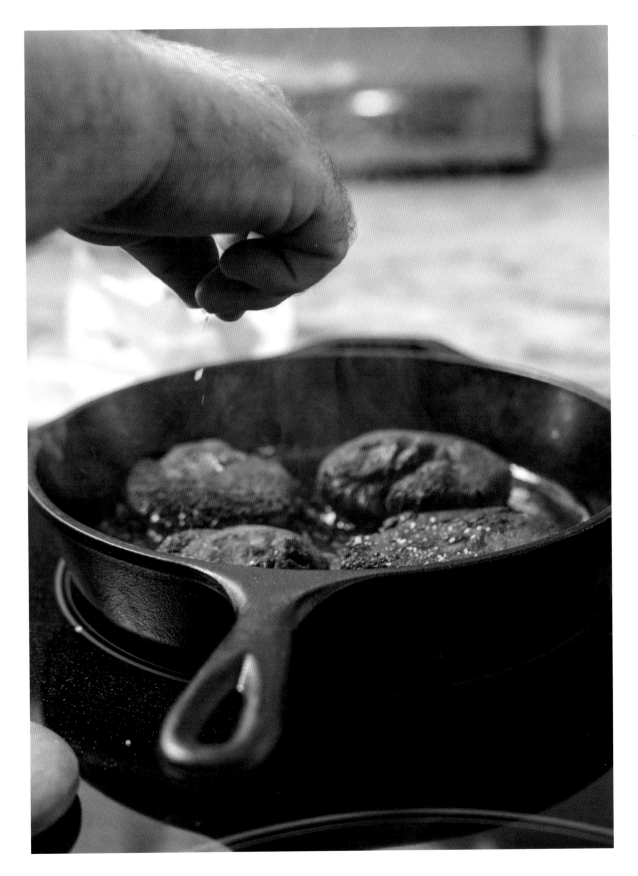

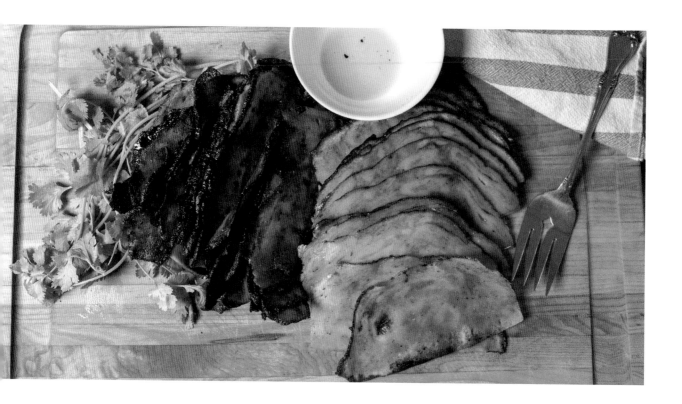

Washed Flour Meat—Oncle Hu Method

Seitan is such a versatile meat replacement. There are so many versions of this pure gluten meat that the possibilities are endless. I was inspired to make this recipe after joining a few seitan Facebook groups. Check out the Seitan Appreciation Society at facebook.com/groups/MakingSeitan.

If there are any recipes in this book I feel you should play around with, I would recommend this one!

This is an adaptation of a recipe by a gentleman named Oncle Hu.

This goes best on a sandwich made from two slices of sourdough bread, vegan swiss cheese, and a large spoonful of sauerkraut! You can even whip up a quick vegan Thousand Island.

Mix together

- ½ cup vegan mayo
- 2 tablespoons ketchup
- 1 tablespoon sweet relish
- 2 teaspoons white vinegar or apple cider vinegar
- 2 tablespoons minced red onion
- Pinch of sugar
- Pinch of salt

INGREDIENTS

4½ CUPS BREAD FLOUR

1 TABLESPOON BEETROOT POWDER

1¾ CUPS WATER

½ TEASPOON BLACK PEPPER

½ TEASPOON CORIANDER

½ TEASPOON PAPRIKA

1 TEASPOON GARLIC POWDER

½ TEASPOON ONION

½ TEASPOON MUSTARD POWDER

1 TEASPOON MUSHROOM
    SEASONINGS

½ CUP OLIVE OIL FOR FRYING

½ CUP RED WINE

¼ CUP SOY SAUCE

DIRECTIONS

- Make dough ball using flour and water. Add beetroot powder to dye dough pinkish red. I make mine in a stand mixer, but you can mix and knead by hand. Knead dough ball until it is firm and bouncy.
- Let rest in a bowl, covered in cold water, for at least an hour.
- After an hour, replace the water and start kneading again in the bowl. You are going to knead in this water until the water turns to a thin buttermilk-like or watery milk appearance. It will be pinkish now because of the beetroot powder. After the first wash, your water will be a thick pink color; dump out the water and wash a second time. You may need to repeat this one more time. But do not over-wash, as you want some remaining starch left in the dough. Look for starchy clumps throughout. The first time I made this, I didn't wash enough.
- Now is time to play with your dough. Stretch, pull, and mangle your dough. This is stretching out the gluten to create strands of gluten. Add in the seasonings and knead together to incorporate.
- Let rest covered for 1 hour.
- Fill skillet with frying oil and heat on a medium heat. Add gluten to skillet and fry, continually flipping, until dark brown on both sides.
- Once desired color has been reached, remove skillet from heat and allow oil to soak up into gluten. Once the pan has cooled, return to the heat and add wine and soy sauce. Cover and allow to simmer for 40 minutes, flipping throughout.
- Wrap and refrigerate overnight.
- You can now fry for a second time, whole, or slice thin and fry individual pieces. I like to slice then fry in a bit more oil, wine, and soy sauce for flavor.

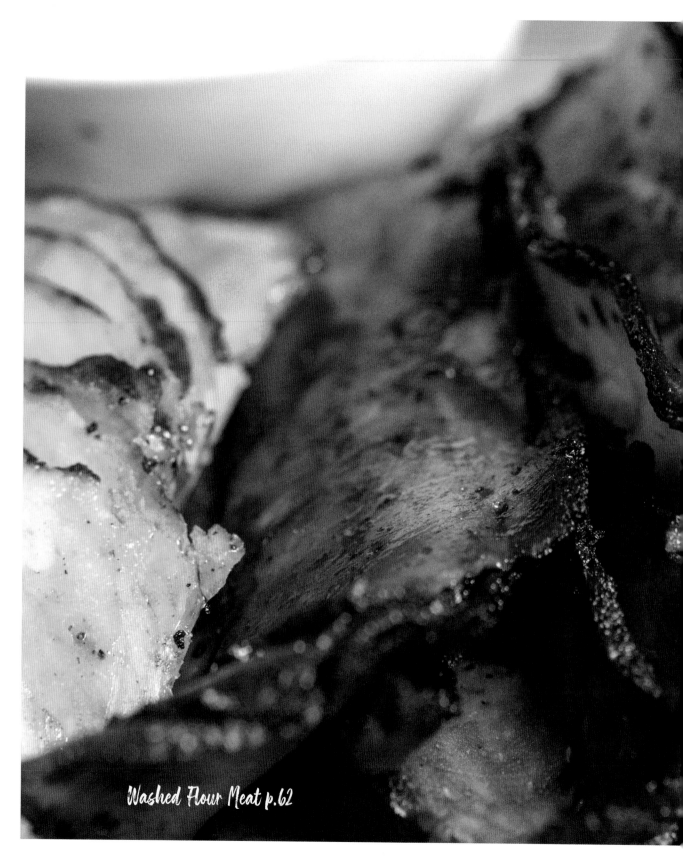

Washed Flour Meat p.62

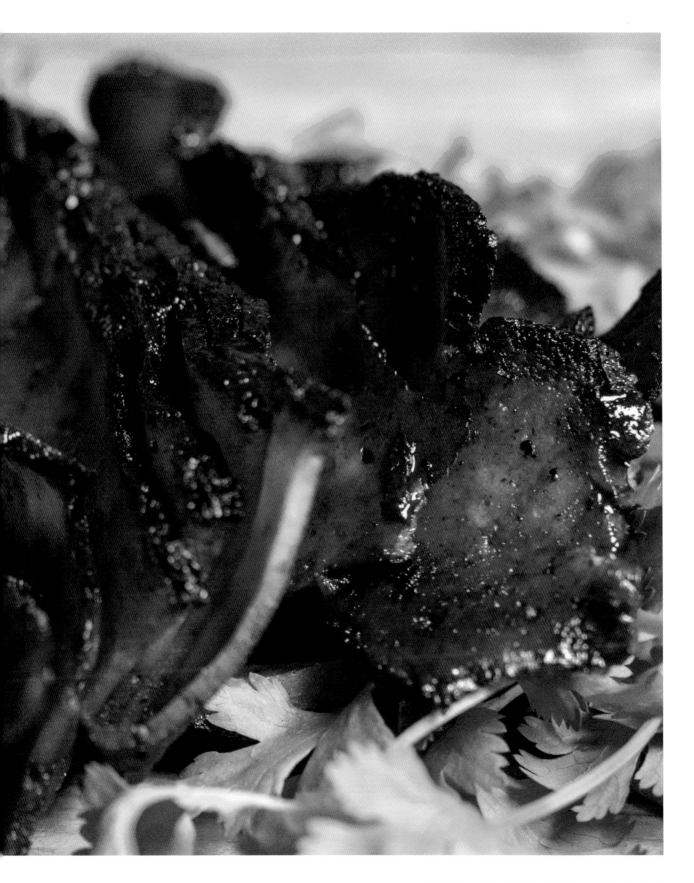

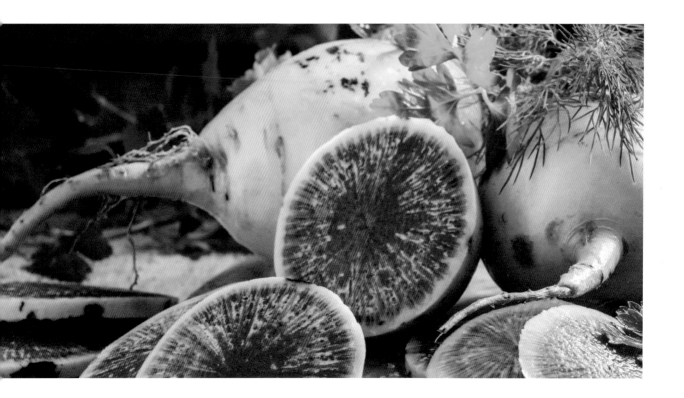

Radish Roast Beef

Another recipe inspired by the incredible chef at Ducks Eatery, Will Horowitz. After watching a wild video where Will made a mind-blowing prosciutto out of a radish, I was inspired to mess with this radish. In one of my earlier tests, I was trying to make it a little more meaty-tasting and ended up coming up with a very roast-beef-like taste and texture. So, I had to run with it. I would love to smoke this like Will did in his prosciutto recipe, or even throw it on a grill low and slow-basting with the flavoring from this recipe. The possibilities are endless.

Try adding some sugars to this to get caramelization, or even using a touch of blackstrap molasses to add that iron-like taste you get from real meat.

You will need two things to make this radish roast beef sandwich whole: horseradish and a 50-50 mix of ketchup and BBQ sauce with a drop of hot sauce!

INGREDIENTS

2 WATERMELON RADISHES WASHED

1 EGG REPLACER

1 TEASPOON BLACK PEPPER

½ TEASPOON GARLIC POWDER

½ TEASPOON LIQUID SMOKE

2 POUNDS KOSHER SALT

BRINE

1½ CUPS WATER

¼ CUP SOY SAUCE

¼ RICE VINEGAR

¼ CUP OLIVE OIL

½ TEASPOON LIQUID SMOKE

½ TEASPOON SMOKED PAPRIKA

½ TEASPOON GARLIC POWDER

½ TEASPOON ONION POWDER

½ TEASPOON BLACK PEPPER

1 TEASPOON MARMITE OR
     NUTRITIONAL YEAST

1 TEASPOON SALT

DIRECTIONS

- In a large bowl, mix egg replacer, garlic powder, black pepper, and liquid smoke. Rub mixture over radish, making sure it is fully coated and that seasonings are "pressed" into skin.
- Preheat oven to 425°F.
- Fill the bottom of a small baking dish with salt, place radish in baking dish, then cover completely in salt.
- Bake in oven for 45 minutes. Remove from oven when done, remove from salt and remove excess salt.
- Slice radish in half and allow to cool while prepping marinade.
- Add all your brine ingredients to a saucepan over medium heat. Bring to a boil, then remove from heat.
- Carefully slice radish on mandoline slicer, and place in glass jar. Cover with brine and place covered in refrigerator overnight.
- Next day, place radish into steamer and steam covered for 30 minutes.
- Enjoy on its own or in a sandwich.

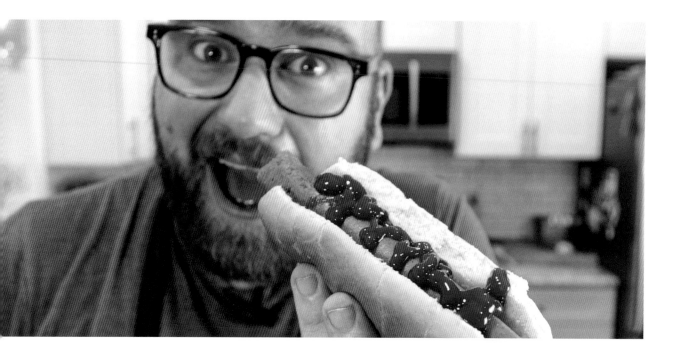

Impossible Vegan Hot Dog

Put on your experimental shoes for this one, because this one is just for fun. I dreamt of creating a meatier, more hot dog-like veggie dog. Now, I don't want to sway you away from your favorite veggie dog, or even the infamous carrot dog that everyone likes to talk about, but this is a new kind of veggie dog. This is a veggie dog that is made more like your traditional hot dog. We are going to start with our TVP burger recipe, or any store-bought burger replacement, and turn it into a vegan real beef hot dog.

When I first tried it, I used store-bought plant-based meat and it came out incredible. I didn't grind it fully into a paste, so the texture wasn't perfect and the color was a little off, but the taste was awesome. I can't wait to see what you come up with after experimenting with this one! Getting the color just right or adding a variety of seasonings to these, to make them totally different hot dogs! It's going to be so great!

Toast the bun and top this the way any hot dog needs to be topped!

My favorite is a chunky hot dog chili sauce!
- 1 cup TVP
- ½ cup ketchup
- 1 tablespoon BBQ sauce
- 1 teaspoon hot sauce
- Salt and pepper to taste
- 2 tablespoons olive oil

Hydrate TVP in boiling water for 15 minutes. Drain and press TVP to remove excess liquid.

Heat skillet over a medium heat and add hydrated TVP. Toss to coat with hot oil and cook for a moment to lightly brown. Turn heat to low and add the rest of the ingredients. Stir to coat, then enjoy on hot dog buns!

INGREDIENTS

FOR THIS YOU WILL NEED DOUBLE
THE TEXTURED PROTEIN
BURGER RECIPE (OR 2 POUNDS
OF ANY PLANT-BASED MEAT)

PLASTIC HOT DOG CASING 26MM–
25MM

¼ CUP VERY FINELY MINCED ONION

1 SMALL CLOVE GARLIC (FINELY
CHOPPED)

1 TEASPOON FINELY GROUND
CORIANDER

½ TEASPOON DRIED MARJORAM

¼ TEASPOON GROUND MACE

½ TEASPOON GROUND MUSTARD

1 TEASPOON SMOKED PAPRIKA

1 TEASPOON FINE GROUND WHITE
PEPPER

3 TABLESPOONS EGG REPLACER

1½ TEASPOONS BROWN SUGAR

1 TEASPOON SALT

½ CUP PLANT-BASED MILK

1 TEASPOON KONJAC GUM

1 TABLESPOON KAPPA
CARRAGEENAN

WILL NEED A SAUSAGE STUFFER, OR
MEAT GRINDER WITH STUFFER

DIRECTIONS

- Mix everything together in a large bowl.
- Grind in food processor or meat grinder to a lumpy fine paste (I ground mine three times in a meat grinder). You'll want a little bit of texture, but not much.
- Place mixture in freezer to chill. We want to keep everything as cold as possible to keep the fat separated and not mixed into the TVP.
- Using a plastic hot dog casing, stuff hot dogs with blended mixture and twist to create hot dogs.
- Cook in boiling water 30 minutes, then remove to cool.
- Once hot dogs are cool, untwist and remove casings. The TVP mixture may have expanded, so we want to wait until the dogs are cool and set before we remove them from their casings.
- These can be eaten right away, or they can be grilled, or pan-fried! Do not boil to reheat.

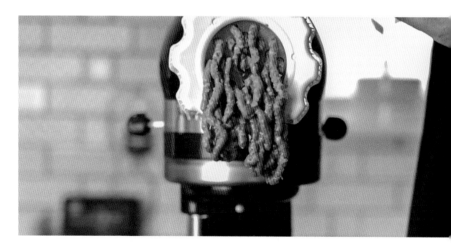

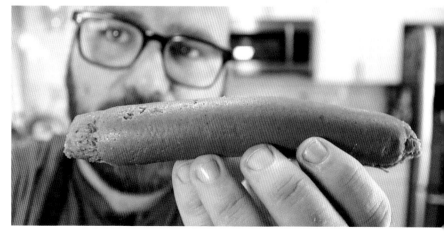

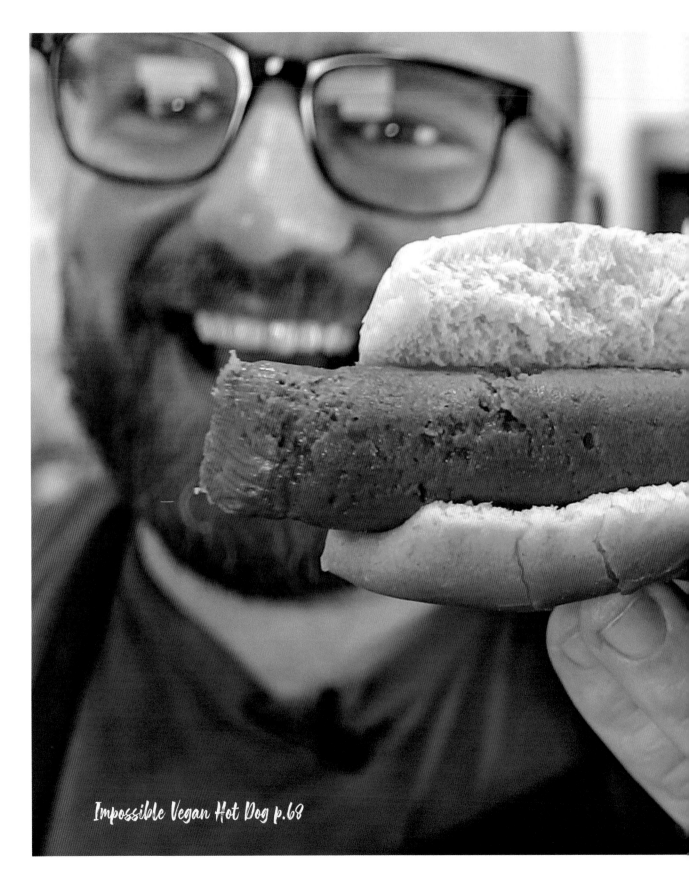

Impossible Vegan Hot Dog p.68

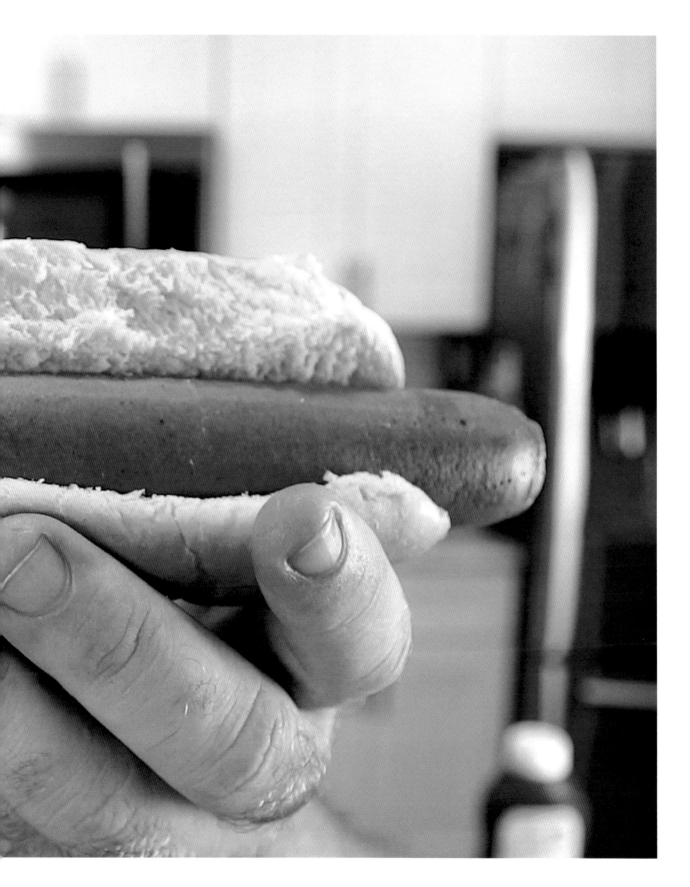

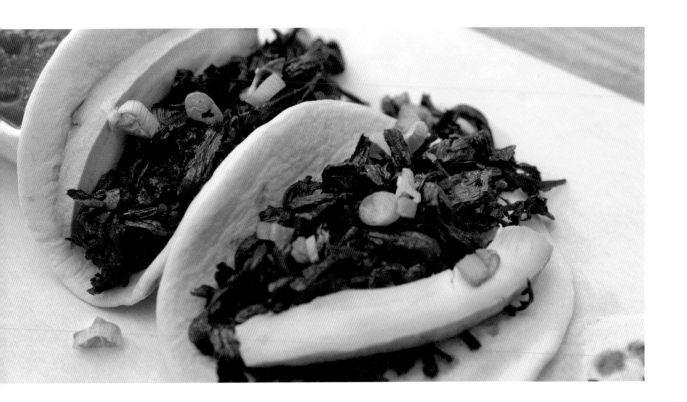

Hibiscus Meat Tacos

This is a traditional Mexican recipe slightly adapted to bring on the meaty flavors. Tacos de Jamaica, as it would be traditionally known, is made from the Jamaica flower, a.k.a. hibiscus. This recipe will provide you with a delicious plant-based ground meat alternative for tacos and a delicious drink by using the water used to hydrate the flower as a tea.

This recipe also includes one of my favorite corn tortilla recipes...they are so easy! You should never buy tortillas!!

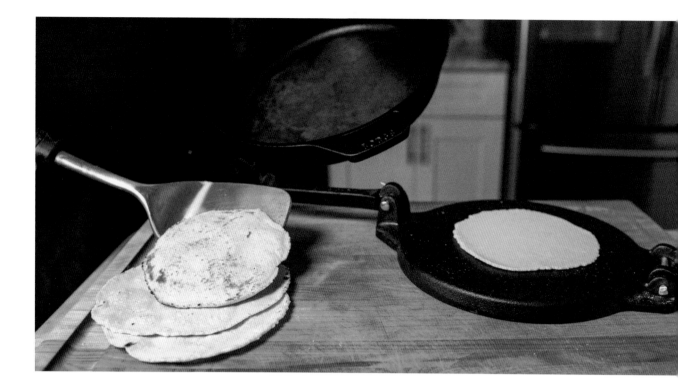

INGREDIENTS

2 CUPS MASA HARINA

1½ CUPS HOT TAP WATER (NOT
HEATED, JUST VERY WARM
FROM A TAP)

PINCH OF SALT

TORTILLA PRESS FOR PERFECT
TACOS, OR YOU CAN USE A
ROLLING PIN

DIRECTIONS

- In a large bowl, add the masa and salt and mix together. Then pour in the hot tap water while mixing.
- This will form a rough flaky dough. Press and knead the dough until you have a smooth dough ball. Cover and let rest for 15 minutes.
- Grab a piece of the dough and roll between your hands to shape a dough ball roughly the size of a golf ball. Slightly larger is okay!
- Using a sheet of plastic wrap, or a ziplock bag cut to fold open, put the dough ball between 2 sheets then press, or put between the two sheets, press with your hand to flatten the dough ball, and use a rolling pin to make small, 4-inch tortillas.
- Heat a pan over high heat. Once the pan is heated, place the tortilla gently onto the pan and allow it to cook for 30 seconds, then flip. You will cook this side for 30 seconds, then flip a last time. Cook for just a moment, then remove from pan. Press and repeat. Keeping cooked corn tortillas covered until finished will give you a perfect soft corn tortilla for the hibiscus tacos.

INGREDIENTS

2 CUPS OF DRIED HIBISCUS
    FLOWER, CLEANED AND WASHED

3 CLOVES OF GARLIC, CHOPPED

½ CUP RED ONION SLICED

2 TABLESPOONS OLIVE OIL

½ TABLESPOON CHILI POWDER

½ TEASPOON GROUND CUMIN

¼ TEASPOON OREGANO

¼ TEASPOON GARLIC POWDER

1 TABLESPOON OLIVE OIL

PINCH OF BLACK PEPPER

PINCH OF SALT

DIRECTIONS

- Fill a large saucepan with your cleaned hibiscus and cover with water. Bring to a boil, then turn heat down to a simmer. Allow to simmer for 10 minutes. After 10 minutes, remove from heat, cover and let rest for 2 hours.
- After 2 hours, strain hibiscus from liquid. You can save this liquid to make a delicious hibiscus tea!
- Heat a large skillet on a medium high heat with olive oil.
- Sauté the onions and garlic, stirring frequently, until they soften and are translucent.
- Add the hibiscus, cooking for a few moments until the flowers darken.
- Add seasonings, stir well to combine, then salt and pepper to taste.
- Build your tacos and enjoy!

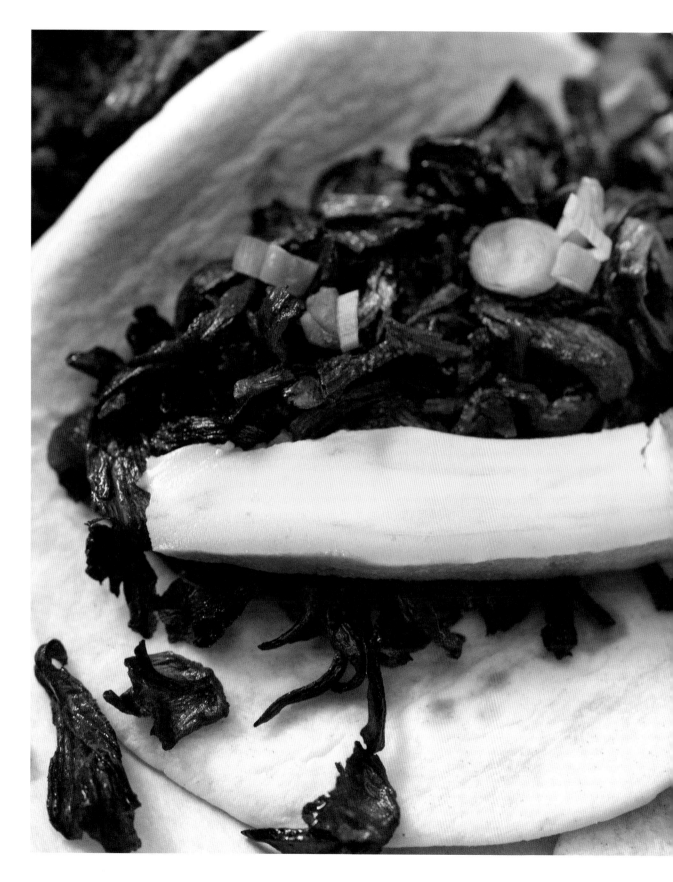

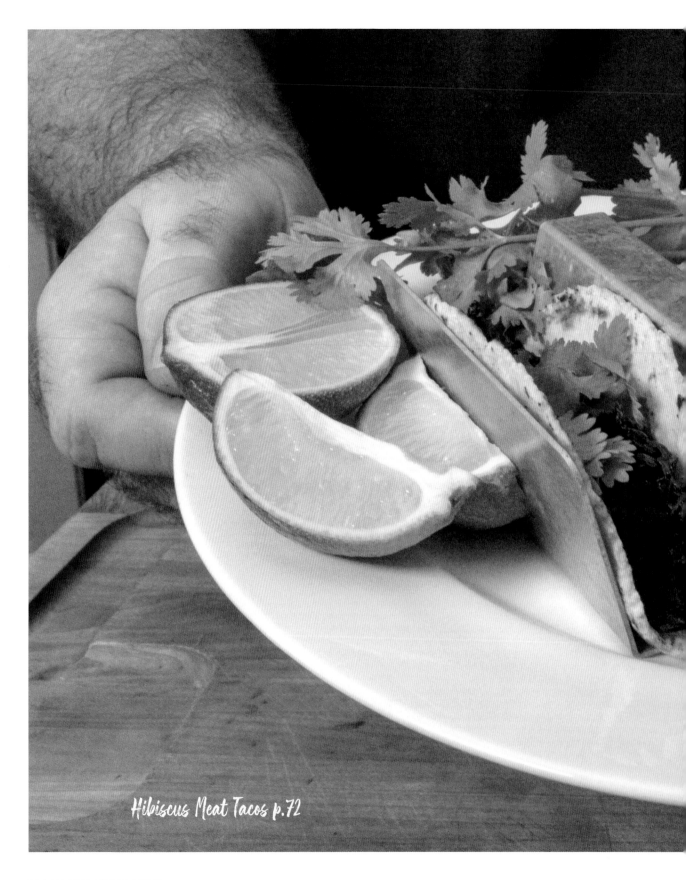

Hibiscus Meat Tacos p.72

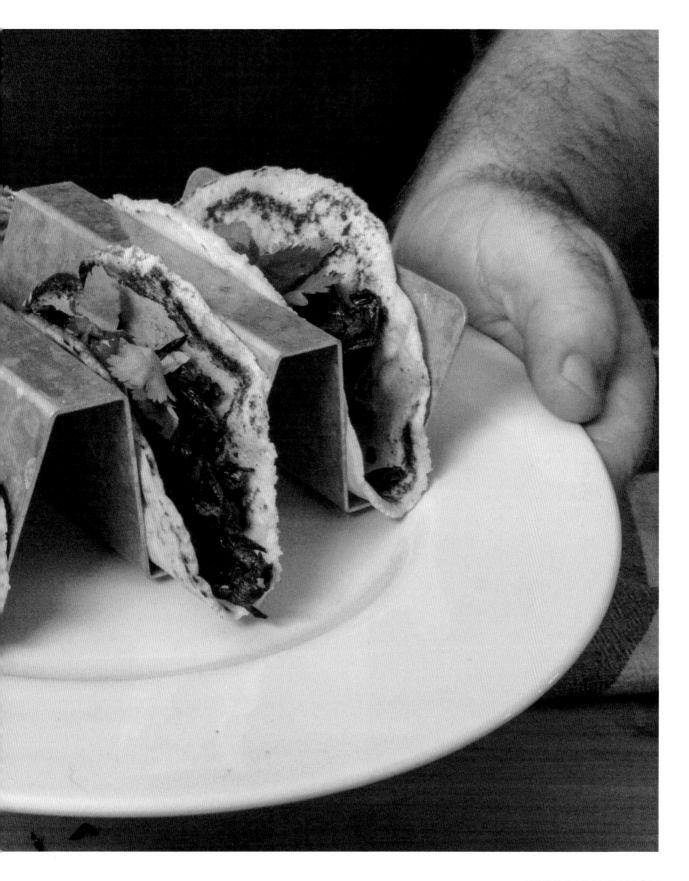

CHICKEN

Or chick-*un* as I annoyingly call it. Chicken is so easily replicated because, as everyone knows, everything tastes like chicken...chick-un. But does it really or is it simply that chicken has a seriously mild taste and most of what you are getting is the texture? I've tried and tried to duplicate that texture...and I've gotten pretty dang close.

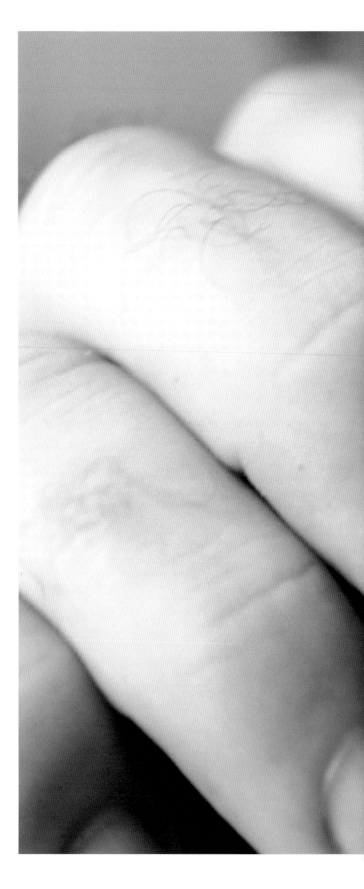

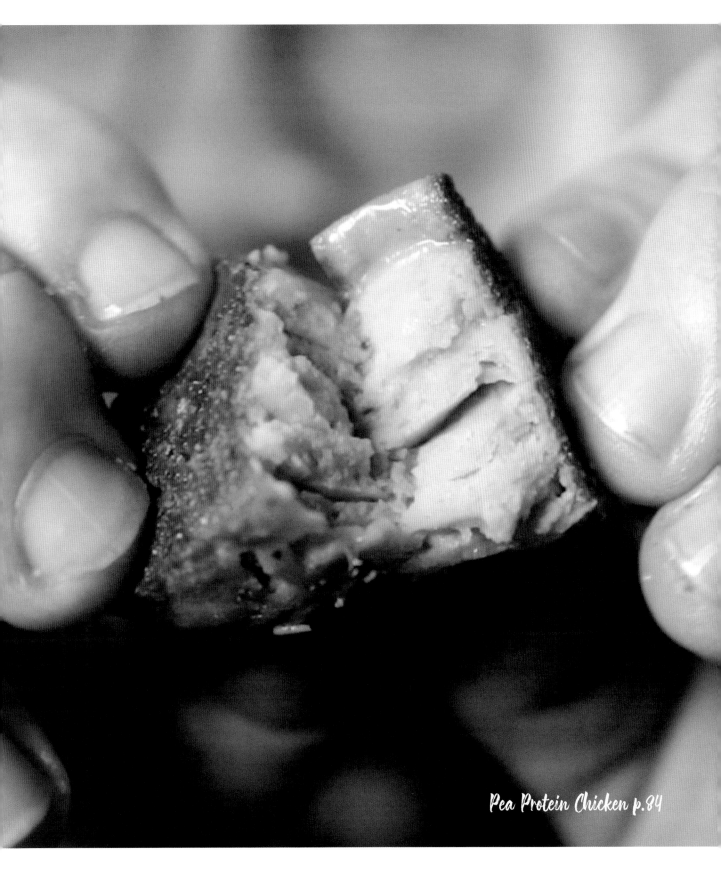

Pea Protein Chicken p.84

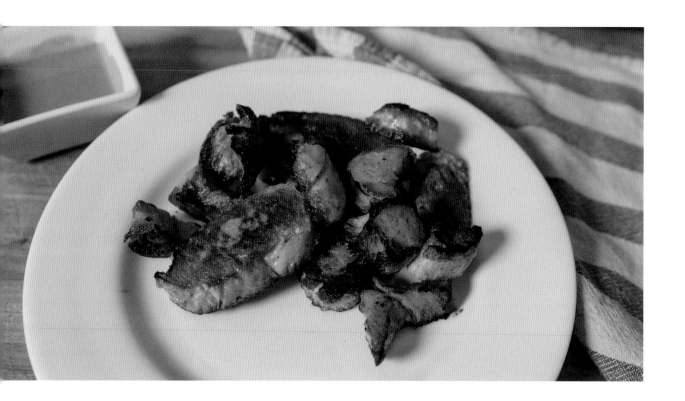

Washed Flour Chicken

The first method used in our chicken (chick-un) chapter using what is known as the washed flour method of seitan. Seitan is made out of pretty much 100 percent gluten. We can make seitan using a vital wheat gluten or by simply "washing" flour. The washed flour method is used a few times in this book. I am including it here as chicken, but experiment with the flavors to create your own unique meat! This is one of my favorites.

This recipe can be adapted for nuggets, strips, or fillets.

Add this chicken to my favorite quick and easy pasta recipe!

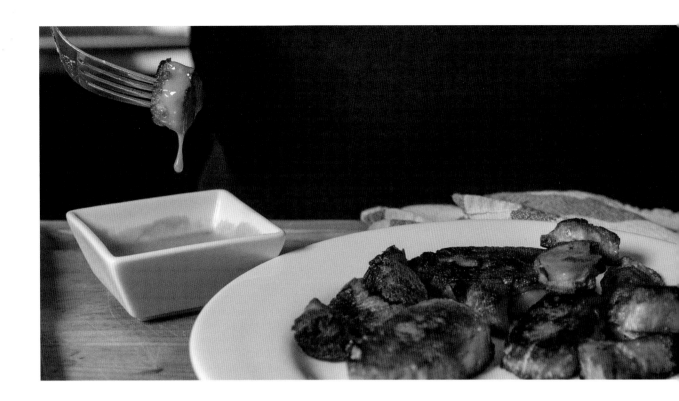

INGREDIENTS

1 28OZ CAN SAN MARZANO
  TOMATOES

3 TABLESPOONS OLIVE OIL

3 TO 6 CLOVES CRUSHED GARLIC

¼ MINCED YELLOW ONION

2 TABLESPOONS TOMATO PASTE

A FEW FRESH BASIL LEAVES

SALT AND PEPPER TO TASTE

DIRECTIONS

- Heat olive oil in a saucepan to a shimmer over a low-medium heat.
- Add garlic and onion and sauté until translucent, then add canned tomatoes. Run a small amount of water into the can and swirl to get all tomato sauce out of can. Bring sauce to a simmer and stir very frequently. Keep covered when not stirring.
- Once you see tomatoes starting to break down into a thicker sauce, add tomato paste, torn-up fresh basil, and salt and pepper to taste.
- Cook sauce for 20 minutes, add chicken, then serve over your favorite pasta!

INGREDIENTS

2½ CUPS BREAD FLOUR

1 CUP WATER

1 TABLESPOON VEGAN CHICKEN
     BROTH SEASONING

DIRECTIONS

- Mix flour and water together to form dough ball, knead until dough is firm. Place dough into bowl and cover in cold water. Let sit for 1 hour.
- After dough as rested, knead dough in water to "wash" away starches. Continue kneading until water is milky. You can then dump water and move to clean water and continue to repeat this step until the water clears. You can wash until perfectly clear water, but I like to stop a little early.
- Your dough should now look stringy, gummy (brain-like).
- Knead the chicken broth seasoning into the dough, then wrap tightly in parchment paper, then wrap in foil.
- Steam in steamer for 45 minutes.
- You can then slice, tear, or cube and treat this as a chicken replacement in any chicken recipe! I like to simply season with a bit of salt and pepper, then pan-sear with a bit of olive oil.

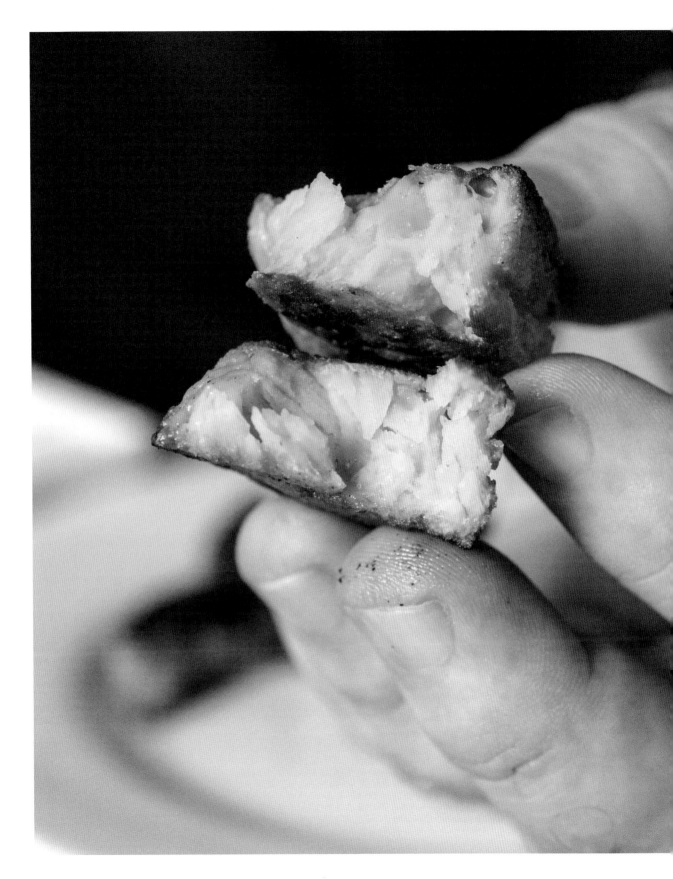

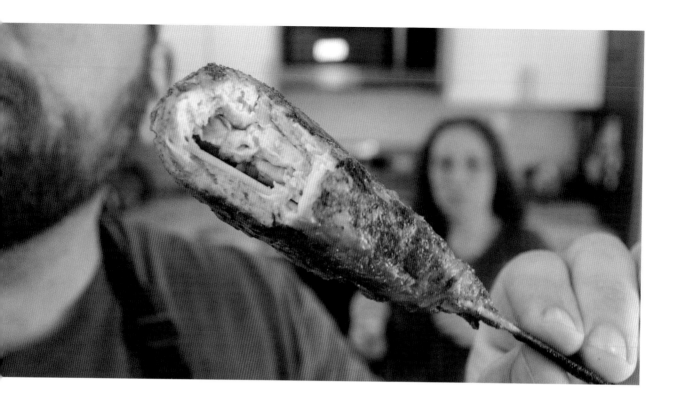

Pea Protein Chicken

By far one of my longest journeys to create a solid meat replacement has to be my pea protein chicken. I started this journey after one of my favorite plant-based chicken replacement suppliers decided to move beyond making chicken and remove their chicken product from the shelves. Pea protein-based chicken is next to impossible to make without using machinery. These large-scale plant-based meat manufacturers make their textured meats using double-screw pressure-heated extruders. These extruders heat, press, and form pea protein, along with flavors, into very chicken-like textured products. After a year of experimenting, this is as close as I could possibly get to that textured extruded plant-based chicken.

I love love love these dipped in some amazing vegan honey mustard... I know honey mustard isn't vegan, but it's really easy to make the vegan version.

- ½ cup Dijon mustard
- ¼ cup agave
- ¼ cup vegan mayo
- 1 teaspoon apple cider vinegar
- ¼ teaspoon paprika

Mix this all up, then dip away!

INGREDIENTS

FOR FAT LAYERS

1½ CUP WATER

1 TEASPOON METHYLCELLULOSE

1 TEASPOON ARROWROOT

2 TABLESPOONS ROOM TEMP LIQUID
    COCONUT OIL

FOR MEAT LAYERS

1 CUP UNFLAVORED PEA PROTEIN

3 TABLESPOONS OF VITAL WHEAT
    GLUTEN

1 TABLESPOON ARROWROOT

1 TEASPOON VEGAN CHICKEN-
    FLAVORED BROTH POWDER OR
    VEGAN CHICKEN BOUILLON

1 TEASPOON METHYLCELLULOSE

½ CUP WATER

¼ CUP WATER

DIRECTIONS

FOR FAT LAYERS

- Pour water into blender and start at slow speed.
- Add methylcellulose and arrowroot. Allow mixture to slightly thicken up.
- While blender is still spinning slowly, drizzle in coconut oil. Start with a slight drip, then slow pour.
- Pour mixture out onto a parchment-paper-lined baking sheet and move to freezer.

FOR MEAT LAYERS

- Add everything from the meat layer into a blender, starting with half a cup of water, and blend until crumbly.
- Add the additional ¼ cup water and blend until everything is well combined.
- Remove from blender and flatten with a roller.
- Cover with parchment paper and allow to rest for 30 minutes.
- After the dough has rested, you can dust with a touch more arrowroot starch and then roll as thin as you can get, resting it if needed. I was able to roll to around ¼-inch thickness.
- Remove fat mixture from freezer once mostly frozen. You should have very thin frozen sheets.
- You will be creating alternating layers of fat and pea protein dough.
- My layers were around 10 inches long by 4 inches wide and 2 inches thick.
- Very tightly wrap in parchment paper, then tightly wrap in foil.
- Fill a large pan or skillet with water and bring to a simmer. Place foil package in water and simmer for 45 minutes.
- Remove from skillet, unwrap, and you can then use this pea protein chicken as you like! Fry it, batter and fry, bake it, season it and grill it!
- This is meant to mimic your plain, unseasoned white chicken meat.

Soy Skin Chicken

Soy skin has so many wild uses! I've used it to make bacon and chicken-wing skin, and now we are looking at this skin to make a whole chicken. Now, this isn't my original idea. Cha Lua Chay is a Vietnamese vegetarian "pork" roll. After trying the original store-bought version, I knew I needed to try to make it...and adapt it to taste like chicken!

My absolute favorite, and I mean favorite, way to use this chicken is by taking it back to its roots and using it in a banh mi!

Find a large thin French bread roll and slice it in half.

Cover with vegan butter, then top sandwich with soy skin chicken, sliced cucumber, fresh cilantro, sliced fresh jalapeno, and pickled daikon and carrot. Then give it a fresh squeeze of siracha.

INGREDIENTS

1-POUND PACKAGE OF SOY SKIN OR
    BEAN CURD SHEETS
1 CAN OF YOUNG GREEN JACKFRUIT
4 CUPS WATER
1 TEASPOON SESAME OIL
1 TABLESPOON MUSHROOM
    SEASONING
1 TEASPOON NUTRITIONAL YEAST
1 TEASPOON VEGAN CHICKEN
    STOCK SEASONING
1 TEASPOON SALT
1 TABLESPOON SOY SAUCE
1 TABLESPOON SUGAR
1 TEASPOON TAPIOCA STARCH

DIRECTIONS

- Add water, oil, mushroom seasoning, chicken stock, nutritional yeast, and jackfruit to large saucepan and bring to a boil.
- Once boiling, turn heat down to a simmer. Slice soy skin into small strips and add to mixture. Simmer until everything is soft.
- Once everything is boiled, strain soy skin and jackfruit in a colander and season with salt, pepper, soy sauce, sugar, and tapioca starch.
- Using parchment paper, wrap half the mixture into a tight log, then wrap in foil very tightly and bind with baker's twine. Repeat for second log.
- The tighter they are wrapped, the better they will come out.
- Let cool and set in refrigerator for around 2 hours.
- Place in steamer basket and steam for an hour.
- Unwrap and slice.

Skinned Cauliflower Wings

I feel like at this point everyone has made cauliflower wings. I think it's a staple in plant-based cooking, but also a staple of any friend who wants to make a plant-based option for their vegan buddy. I've seen cauliflower wings at parties, on platters, and I've even made them for lunch. But you've never had a cauliflower wing like this. This one has a skin!

INGREDIENTS

HEAD OF CAULIFLOWER, CLEANED
    AND SEPARATED INTO FLORETS
SOY MILK OR STORE-BOUGHT
    FROZEN SOY SKIN
5 TEASPOONS VEGAN CHICKEN
    BROTH SEASONING
5 CUPS WATER

SAUCE
2 TABLESPOONS VEGAN BUTTER
¼ CUP FRANKS REDHOT
1 TEASPOON CHIPOTLE TABASCO
1 TABLESPOON MAPLE SYRUP

DIRECTIONS

- Make a chicken broth in saucepan filled with water and vegan chicken broth seasoning. Bring to boil, then add cauliflower florets. Boil for 3 minutes.
- Remove cauliflower from boiling water, then run cold water over it.
- If using store-bought bean curd sheets, place sheet into water to hydrate, then remove and wrap around cauliflower and place on parchment-lined baking sheet.
- If using soy milk, heat soy milk in large nonstick skillet to boil. Once it's boiling, lower heat to a slow simmer and wait until you see a skin develop around the entire surface of the milk. Use a spatula to work around the sides of the skillet to detach skin from skillet, then lift from underneath, wrapping around cauliflower. Place cauliflower on a parchment-lined baking sheet.
- Preheat oven to 450°F.
- Bake "wings" for 25 minutes, flip, then cook for an additional 5 minutes.
- In a saucepan, add all the ingredients for the sauce and whisk together.
- Toss the "wings" in the sauce.

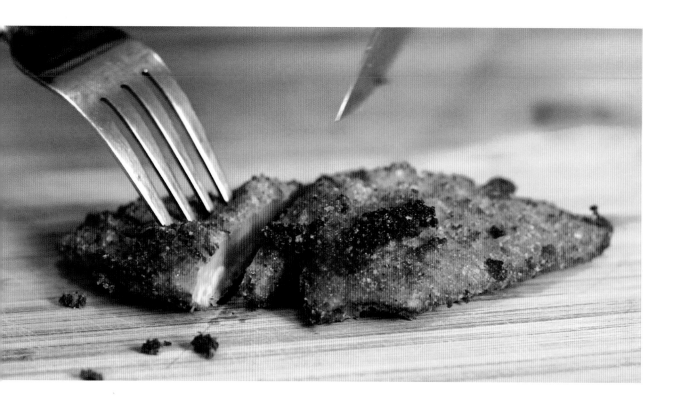

Grapefruit Meat Chicken

Another recipe that has origins outside of the plant-based world is the grapefruit steak. Bistec de Toronja, which means grapefruit steak, originates from Cuba during a dark time. It was originally created out of necessity in the '90s during the Cuban food shortage, when Cubans were looking for ways to use every possible food. I adapted this recipe simply because I do love the idea of less food waste, but also being open to trying something new. This has a unique texture and mild enough taste that it can be flavored and really messed with to create something truly unique. This one might not be for everyone, but if you're open to it, you might be pleasantly surprised.

Throw these in a sandwich with some grilled onions and cilantro, maybe top with a bit of hot sauce, and you will have a mind-blowing sandwich experience… Can you tell how much I like to make sandwiches?!

INGREDIENTS

2 LARGE GRAPEFRUIT

8 CLOVES GARLIC, CRUSHED

2 TEASPOONS BAKING SODA

4 CUPS WATER

2 EGG REPLACEMENT EQUIVALENTS

1 TABLESPOON FRESH PARSLEY,
    MINCED

SALT AND PEPPER TO TASTE

2 CUPS BREADCRUMBS

VEGETABLE OIL TO FRY

DIRECTIONS

- Peel the outer skin of the grapefruit using a speed peeler. Only remove the tough outer layer, leaving the inside white layer known as the pith.
- Slice the grapefruit into quarters, then carefully remove the grapefruit meat! (Enjoy this part on its own.)
- Make small slices around the edges of the curved sides to help the pieces of peel lie flat.
- Fill a bowl with the water, add baking soda and grapefruit peels. Allow to rest in the water for 10 minutes.
- Remove peels and dry with a paper towel. Rub the peels vigorously on both sides with the crushed garlic.
- In a large bowl, prepare your egg replacer, add parsley, salt, and pepper, then whisk. Place breadcrumbs on a plate.
- Heat 1 inch of oil in an iron skillet.
- Dip the peels into the egg replacer mixture, then roll them into the breadcrumbs and fry.

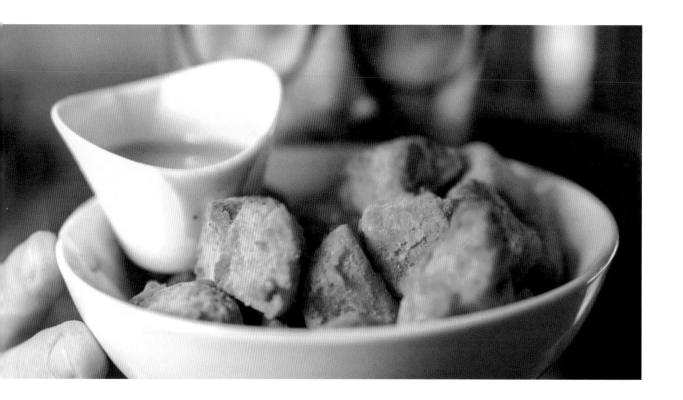

Better Seitan Chicken Nuggets

I absolutely love the texture that seitan gives us, but I also love the texture of textured vegetable protein or TVP. When we combine those two, we end up with a highly textured product that's always reminded me of fast-food chicken. Now, the best part of this chicken is, you can make it seven days a week, even on Sundays. So, let's whip us up some chicken nuggets and some bonus dipping sauce.

My favorite thing about these nuggets is how versatile they are. You can use them in so many different recipes, but all it takes is changing the breading around to turn these into any of your fast-food favorites.

Closed on Sunday Style Chicken Dipping Sauce

- ¼ cup vegan mayo
- 2 tablespoons agave
- 1 tablespoon Dijon mustard
- 1 tablespoon yellow mustard
- 2 tablespoons BBQ sauce

Mix it all together! Dip nuggets in bowl, pour over any chicken sandwich, or just drink it out of the bowl.

INGREDIENTS

- 4 TABLESPOONS VITAL WHEAT GLUTEN
- 1 CUP TVP
- 1 TABLESPOON METHYLCELLULOSE
- 1 TEASPOON XANTHAN GUM
- 1 TABLESPOON TAPIOCA STARCH
- 1 TEASPOON VEGAN CHICKEN BROTH BOUILLON OR POWDER
- 1 CUP WATER
- ½ TEASPOON SOY SAUCE
- ½ TEASPOON WHITE DISTILLED VINEGAR
- ¼ TEASPOON MARMITE
- 1 TABLESPOON LIGHT OIL

DIRECTIONS

- Place the TVP into a blender and pulse briefly. Don't overblend, you just want smaller chunks of TVP.
- Mix all dry ingredients together and mix wet ingredients separately, then mix the two together.
- Mix together first to make sure all ingredients are combined.
- Remove from bowl and knead by hand. When kneading, knead flat, then fold layer over top, continue in this flattening, then folding, kneading method until the "chicken" feels firm.
- Lightly oil a sheet of foil, then wrap chicken very tight.
- Steam "chicken" in a steamer basket for 40–60 minutes (it'll feel very firm).
- Tear chicken into nugget-sized pieces. You should get around 12.

NUGGET BREADING (CLOSED ON SUNDAY STYLE BREADING)

INGREDIENTS

- ¾ CUP BREADCRUMBS
- ¾ CUP ALL-PURPOSE FLOUR
- 2 TABLESPOONS POWDERED SUGAR
- 2 TEASPOONS KOSHER SALT
- ½ TEASPOON BLACK PEPPER
- ½ TEASPOON CHILI POWDER
- 6 TABLESPOONS EGG REPLACER
- 1 CUP PLANT-BASED MILK (SEE MILK FAVORITES)
- 1 TABLESPOON PICKLE JUICE

DIRECTIONS

- Mix dry ingredients together and wet ingredients together in two separate bowls.
- Place nuggets in wet mix and allow to rest for 10 minutes.
- Then dip in dry mix.
- Place dredged nuggets on rack and allow mixture to soak in.
- Fill a large iron skillet or Dutch oven with frying oil, at least 3 inches of oil. Vegetable oil or peanut oil works well. Heat to between 350 and 360°F.
- Fry in small batches, keeping the oil temp between 350 and 360°F.
- When patties are a deep golden brown, remove them to a wire rack.
- Lightly salt to taste.

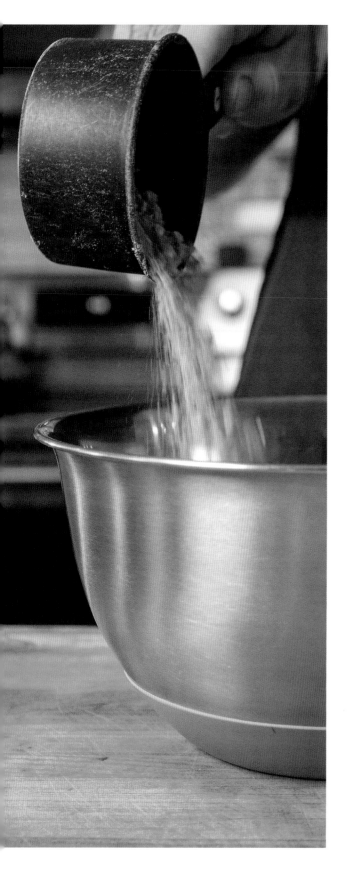

The Chicken Nugget

Now, I love experimenting, and I wanted to include some of those experiments in the book. Not every experiment is bad until it gets better. The recipe on the previous page makes a chicken nugget with the combination of TVP and gluten. This was an earlier version of that recipe, without the vital wheat gluten.

You end up with a more tender, juicier nugget that lacks some of the bite. Experiment to see what works for you. This is also a recipe that, with a few changes, can be made gluten-free.

Did you see the recipe I made earlier for the vegan honey mustard? You will want that recipe for this! It's on page 84 with the pea protein chicken! Go make it now!

INGREDIENTS

CHICKEN

½ CUP WATER

½ CUP TVP

½ TABLESPOON MUSHROOM
    SEASONING

½ TABLESPOON NUTRITIONAL YEAST

1 TEASPOON VEGAN CHICKEN
    BROTH SEASONING

1 TABLESPOON METHYLCELLULOSE,
    HIGH-VISCOSITY

2 TABLESPOONS PEA PROTEIN

2 TEASPOONS XANTHAN GUM

1 TSP COCONUT OIL

SALT AND PEPPER

FOR BREADING

DRY INGREDIENTS

½ CUP FLOUR

¼ CUP CORN STARCH

½ TABLESPOON SALT

½ TEASPOON SUGAR

¼ TEASPOON WHITE PEPPER

¼ TEASPOON ONION POWDER

½ TEASPOON BLACK PEPPER

WET INGREDIENTS

1 TABLESPOON FLOUR

1 TABLESPOON CORN STARCH

½ TEASPOON SUGAR

½ CUP COLD SPARKLING WATER

1 EGG REPLACER

PINCH OF SALT

VEGETABLE OIL FOR FRYING

DIRECTIONS

- Mix all ingredients from the chicken list together in large bowl, cover, and let rest for 30 minutes.
- Once TVP chicken mixture is hydrated, form into chicken nugget shapes, cover, and freeze until firm.
- Mix dry breading ingredients together, and in a separate bowl mix the wet ingredients together.
- Heat oil in large skillet or Dutch oven to 350°F; remove nuggets from freezer. Dip nuggets in dry batter to coat, then dip into wet batter, then back into the dry batter. Let rest on wire rack for 5 minutes.
- Fry in oil in small batches, to not overcrowd, until light golden brown, constantly turning.

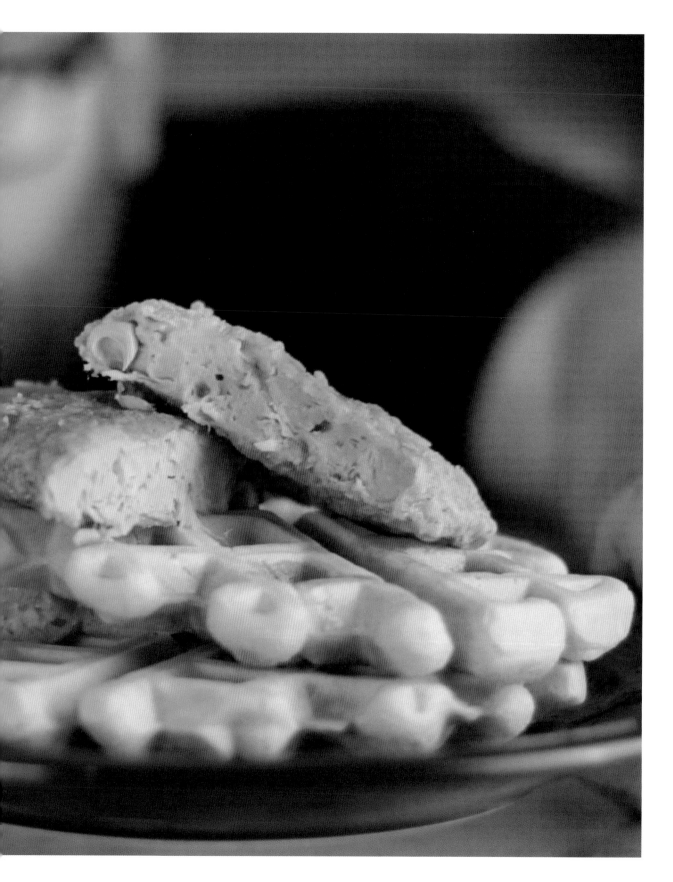

Fried Jackfruit Chicken (Nuggets or Patties)

Jackfruit has always been at the top of my list of my favorite meaty plants. Its texture when unripe is so close to pulled pork, it's uncanny. But that pulled pork texture is really what got my wheels turning. We've used jackfruit earlier in this book, but this is the first recipe where it is the star of the show. This recipe, like most of our other chick-un recipes, can be made as nuggets or patties and is incredibly versatile. I've used it for chicken and waffles (bonus waffle recipe below). I've also used it to make a Nashville hot jackfruit. You can throw on some vegan parm or white cheese to make a pretty killer vegan parm or fry it, chop it up, and toss it into your favorite salad. This is by far one of my favorites.

I know when I make fried chick-un breast, the one thing I always thick of is chicken and waffles! I don't know why... Haha, but I'm telling you, this. Is. Good! You'll slow-clap after your first bite of this combo. I promise!

INGREDIENTS

1 CUP FLOUR

1 TABLESPOON SUGAR

2 TEASPOONS BAKING POWDER

PINCH OF SALT

2 TABLESPOONS EGG REPLACER
(SEE EGG REPLACERS FOR CHOICES)

¾ CUP PLANT-BASED MILK

¼ CUP VEGETABLE OIL

½ TEASPOON VANILLA EXTRACT

DIRECTIONS

- Mix dry ingredients together well.
- Then add wet ingredients, then mix all together.
- Allow mixture to rest for 10 minutes.
- Heat waffle iron and coat with nonstick spray or brush lightly with oil.
- Cook in waffle iron and enjoy some serious vegan waffles!

INGREDIENTS

2 20-OZ. CANS YOUNG GREEN
    JACKFRUIT
1½ CUPS WATER
1 VEGAN CHICKEN BOUILLON OR
    1 TABLESPOON CHICKEN-
    FLAVORED BROTH POWDER
2 TABLESPOONS NUTRITIONAL YEAST
2 TABLESPOONS PROTEIN POWDER
    (PEA PROTEIN OR FAVA BEAN
    PROTEIN)
1 TABLESPOON METHYLCELLULOSE

DRY BATTER (ANY OF YOUR
FAVORITE BATTERS WILL WORK
WITH THIS RECIPE. DRY BATTER OR
WET BATTER)
1 CUP FLOUR
½ TEASPOON PAPRIKA
½ TEASPOON CHILI POWDER
½ TEASPOON GARLIC POWDER
½ TEASPOON BLACK PEPPER

WET BATTER
4 TABLESPOONS EGG REPLACER
1 CUP PLANT-BASED MILK
WANNA MAKE THIS HOT? USE
    1–4 TABLESPOONS OF YOUR
    FAVORITE HOT SAUCE
VEGETABLE OIL FOR FRYING

DIRECTIONS

- Drain and wash the jackfruit.
- Separate seeds and break jackfruit apart from their stem corners. You can squeeze the edge and the seeds will pop out of their shells. Discard the seeds.
- Bring the water to a boil along with bouillon and nutritional yeast. Once water is at a rolling boil, add jackfruit, lower heat to a simmer, and stir. Boil until less than half of the liquid remains.
- Remove from heat.
- Add protein powder and mix.
- Allow mixture to cool below 120°F.
- Add methylcellulose, mix together.
- Lay out a shoebox-sized piece of plastic wrap and drop a quarter of the jackfruit mixture onto it.
- You can make 4 large patties with this, or around a dozen smaller, nugget-sized pieces.
- Wrap tightly and form into chicken breast shape.
- Place in freezer and allow to freeze. You can freeze until ready to use.
- Fill a large iron skillet or Dutch oven with frying oil, at least 3 inches of oil. Vegetable oil or peanut oil works well. Heat to 350–360°F.
- Using two separate bowls, mix dry batter ingredients together in one bowl and wet batter ingredients together in another large bowl.
- Dip frozen patties into dry mix, then into wet mix, then back into dry mix.
- Place covered patties on a rack for 10–15 minutes.
- Then fry patties two at a time, keeping the oil temp between 350 and 360°F.
- When patties are a deep golden brown, remove them to a wire rack.
- Lightly salt to taste.

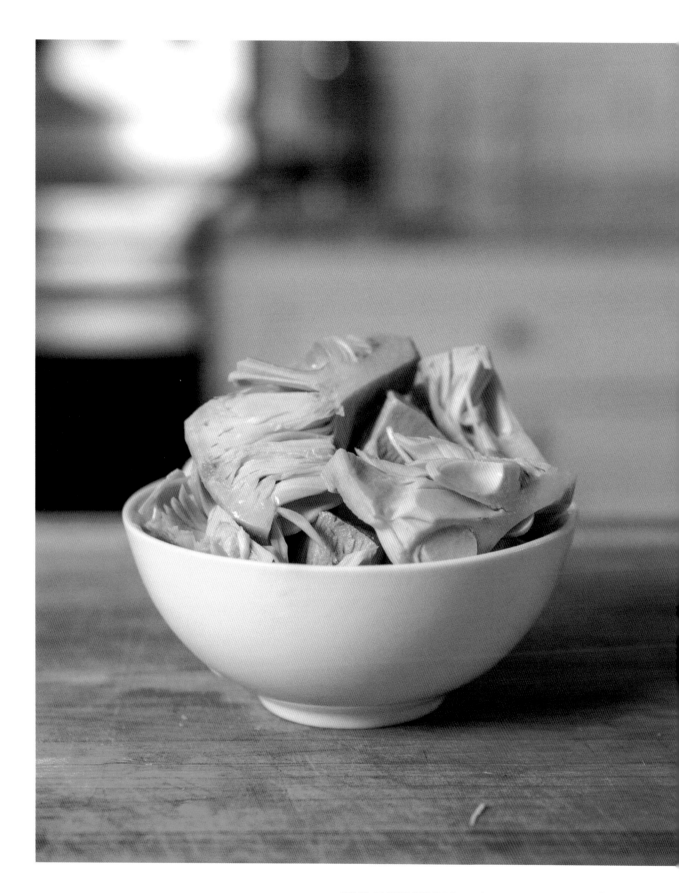

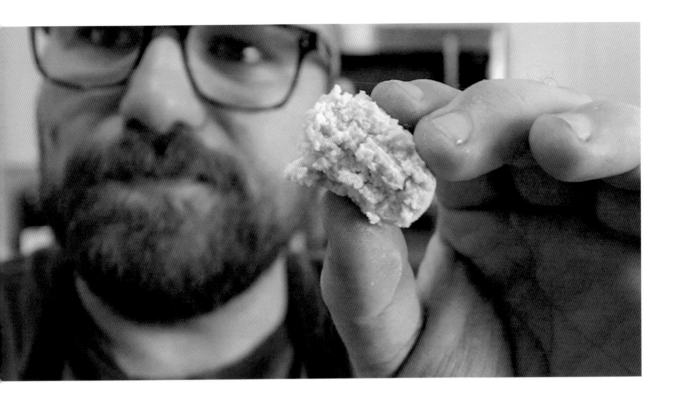

Twice-Frozen Tofu Chicken Strips

The best thing about tofu is something you've probably already heard. It can taste like whatever you cook it in.

Sounds a little like chicken, doesn't it? This recipe was originally inspired by a visit to one of my local favorite Chinese restaurants that's now closed, eating one of my favorites, General Tso Tofu. This is my version of that recipe, but there was also some inspiration from another favorite creator of mine, Mary's Test Kitchen.

For some reason, any time I make these tofu chicken strips, I always want to top them with my favorite chili glaze sauce! You can't beat it, and it's incredibly simple to make.

CHILI GLAZE SAUCE

INGREDIENTS

½ CUP SOY SAUCE

¼ CUP BROWN SUGAR

¼ CUP SESAME OIL

5 GARLIC CLOVES, MINCED

½ CUP MIRIN

½ TEASPOON RED PEPPER FLAKES

2 TEASPOONS CORNSTARCH

1 TABLESPOON WATER

DIRECTIONS

- In a small saucepan, mix together everything except the cornstarch and water and bring to a slow simmer. In a separate bowl, whisk the cornstarch and water together. Now whisk the corn starch slurry into the simmering soy glaze mixture to desired thickness!
- Now, once you make your fried tofu nuggets or strips, you can cover them with this rich, thick sweet glaze sauce!

CHICKEN STRIPS

INGREDIENTS

1 PACKAGE OF MEDIUM OR FIRM TOFU

1 TEASPOON VEGAN CHICKEN
    BROTH POWDER

¼ CUP HOT/WARM WATER

BREADING

WET INGREDIENTS

1 CUP CASHEW MILK OR PEA
    PROTEIN MILK

1 TEASPOON LEMON JUICE

1 TABLESPOON FRANKS REDHOT

5 TABLESPOONS LIQUID EGG
    REPLACER OR 2 EGG EQUIVALENT

DRY INGREDIENTS

1 CUP FLOUR

2 TEASPOONS PAPRIKA

1 TEASPOON GARLIC POWDER

1 TABLESPOON CAYENNE PEPPER

3 TEASPOONS PEPPER

PINCH OF SALT

VEGETABLE OIL FOR FRYING

DIRECTIONS

- To start with this recipe, we want to double-freeze our tofu! Do not open your tofu; throw it in the freezer. Allow it to freeze solid, then remove from the freezer to completely thaw. Once thawed, throw back in the freezer and keep frozen until you are ready to use.
- Remove frozen tofu from freezer and allow to fully thaw, open, drain, and dry your tofu, then, using a tofu press or a few cutting boards or cookbooks (not this one), press your tofu to remove excess water. Double-frozen tofu is easier to press but can also start to break apart. Make sure you give your tofu plenty of drying time, as the drier the tofu is, the better it will be.
- Once tofu is ready, get three separate bowls. Mix hot water and chicken broth mix in one bowl, wet batter ingredients in a second, and dry batter ingredients in the third bowl.
- Heat oil in a large skillet or Dutch oven to 350°F.
- Tear tofu gently into desired sizes, briefly dip in chicken broth, then dry batter, then wet batter, then dry batter, and place on a wire rack or plate.
- Fry tofu strips in oil until golden brown and remove to wire rack or paper towel to dry.
- Salt to taste.

EGGS

(ARE EGGS MEAT?)

What came first, the chicken or the egg? Well, in this book the chicken did. This next chapter is all about making the incredible edible vegan egg. There are quite a few methods to make a great vegan egg and we are going to start with one of the easiest and move our way into some really great molecular gastronomy.

Grab your black salt and let's make some eggs.

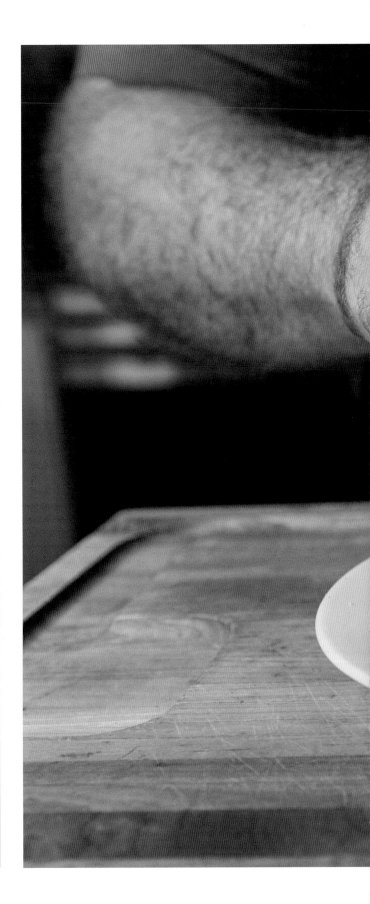

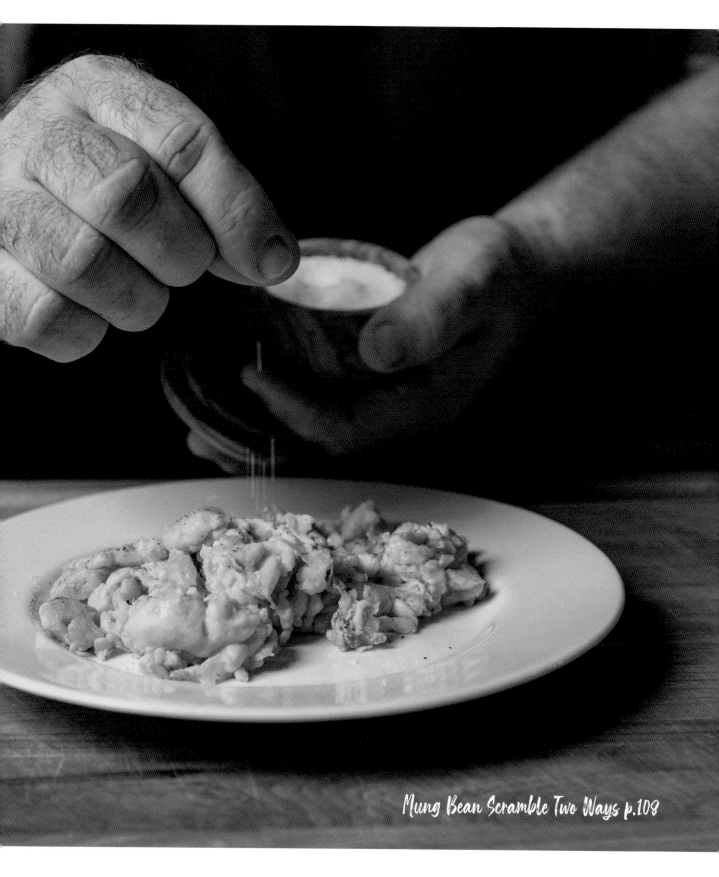

Mung Bean Scramble Two Ways p.108

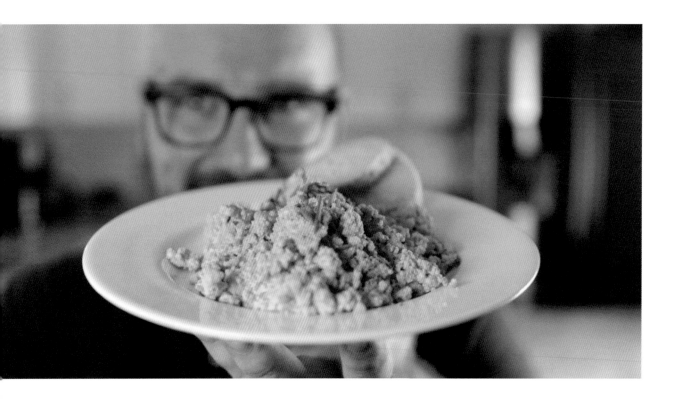

Better Tofu Scramble

Our first plant-based egg on this list is an egg everyone knows, the tofu scramble. With most tofu scrambles, you have individual bits of tofu broken up, flavored, and colored to look like egg. The taste is there, it's pretty good, but I always found the texture to be off. That's why I wanted to work on making tofu scramble better!

I love scrambles so much, and I love scrambles and toast. I just don't think there is a better pair, except when you add in avocado toast.

Toast a slice of sourdough bread, and butter that sucker with a bit of vegan butter.

Mash up a large avocado and mix in 2 teaspoons agave, a pinch of crushed red peppers, and a pinch of kosher salt. Spread the avocado mixture on the toast, then top that hipster toast off with a big scoop of the better tofu scramble.

INGREDIENTS

1 BLOCK OF FIRM TOFU

1 TEASPOON TURMERIC

1 TEASPOON OF BLACK SALT

¼ TEASPOON VEGAN CHICKEN
    BOUILLON

1 TEASPOON NUTRITIONAL YEAST

SALT AND PEPPER TO TASTE

½ CUP CASHEW MILK

½ TEASPOON KAPPA CARRAGEENAN

DIRECTIONS

- Drain tofu, then place in a mixing bowl and mash using a fork or potato masher.
- Whisk cashew milk with turmeric, black salt, chicken bouillon, and kappa carrageenan.
- Add milk mixture to tofu and mix well. Allow to rest for 10 minutes.
- Lightly oil a nonstick skillet, then add tofu scramble mixture and cook over a high heat.
- Bring the mixture to a simmer and cook mixture down to desired consistency.
- Remove from heat and let rest for 15 minutes. Lightly scramble mixture.
- Add salt and pepper, then serve.

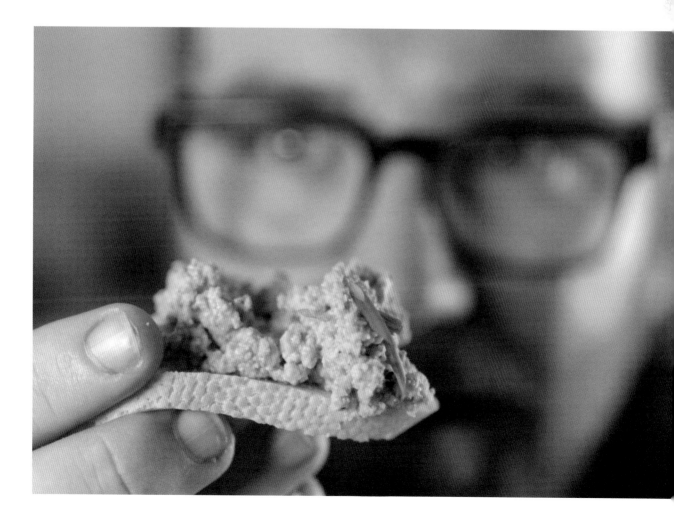

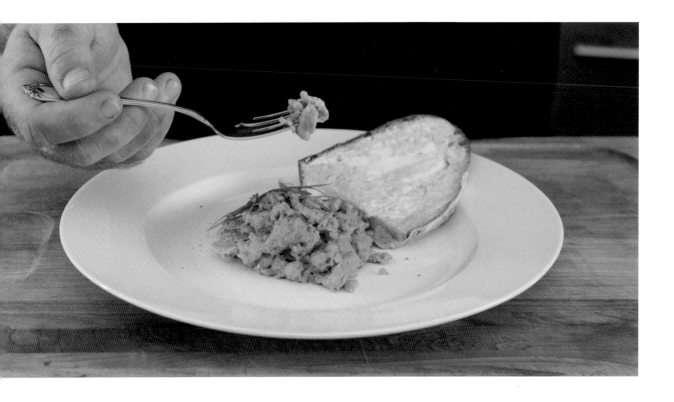

Pumpkin Seed Egg

We are going to quickly move away from the normal plant-based egg and move into something I found incredibly unique. I would never have imagined that a pumpkin seed would taste eggy, but with a few tweaks and a few twists, it's totally possible. This vegan scramble is so incredibly egg-like, people will double-take when you tell them it came from a pumpkin seed.

Eat this one just as it is! Scramble it, maybe toss in some of your favorite vegan cheeses. Enjoy this as a wildly eggy scrambled egg.

INGREDIENTS

10 OZ RAW PUMPKIN SEEDS

2¼ CUP WATER

1 TEASPOON TURMERIC

½ TEASPOON GARLIC POWDER

1 TEASPOON BLACK SALT

1 TABLESPOON OLIVE OIL PER
    "SCRAMBLE"

DIRECTIONS

- Cover pumpkin seeds with cool water and let sit overnight.
- Drain and wash pumpkin seeds under water to remove skin. Remove as much of the skin as possible.
- Add pumpkin seeds to blender along with 2¼ cups water and blend until very smooth.
- Add flavorings and blend to combine.
- Place in the refrigerator overnight.
- Add olive oil to nonstick skillet and place on medium high heat. Pour in desired egg amount.
- Allow to cook through on one side. When you see the top slightly dry, start to slowly scramble.
- Season with salt and pepper or your favorite egg toppings.

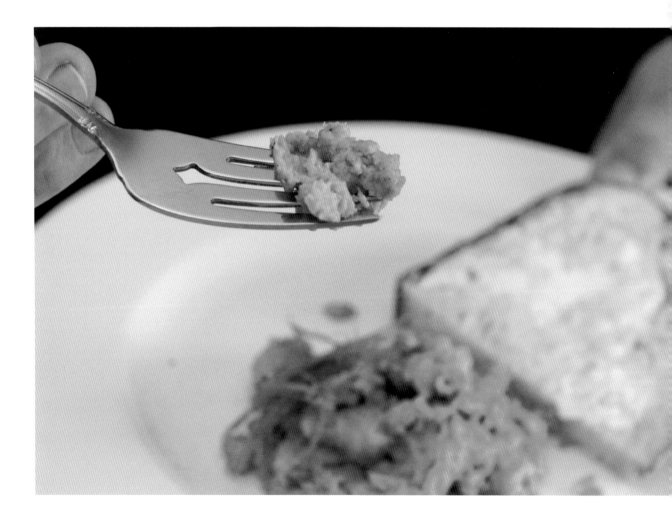

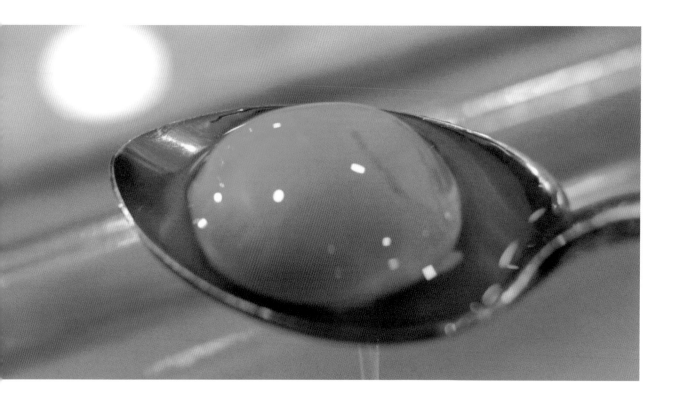

The Secret Tomato "Egg" Yolk Recipe

I love breaking out the science kit when I'm cooking, and this egg moves into that territory. This recipe was inspired by the chefs at Crossroads Kitchen. After seeing a few videos people shared of their Crossroads Kitchen egg yolks, I knew I had to try to make it. A lot of what I saw I knew how to do, and a lot already made sense in terms of what would work to get a tomato to taste like an egg yolk. Yellow tomatoes themselves are fairly mild and are loaded with glutamates, just like egg yolks are. With a few tweaks of the flavor, I knew it would be easy to get the tomato to resemble an egg's taste; the trick was tackling some old molecular gastronomy tricks to get that tomato into a yolk shape that would "pop."

INGREDIENTS

2 LARGE YELLOW TOMATOES

3 CUPS DISTILLED WATER

5 TEASPOONS SODIUM ALGINATE

1 TABLESPOON CALCIUM CHLORIDE

3 + 1 TABLESPOON OLIVE OIL

1 TEASPOON MUSTARD POWDER

2 TABLESPOONS NUTRITIONAL
    YEAST

2 TEASPOONS BLACK SALT

DIRECTIONS

- Make your alginate gel first. You will want to make this around 4 hours in advance, or the night before. Start with 3 cups distilled water in a blender spinning at a slow speed, then slowly add sodium alginate. This will create a gel.
- Pour the gel into a shallow dish, cover, and refrigerate to rest. We are resting it to remove air bubbles. If you do not remove air bubbles, you will get air bubbles in your egg yolk casing.
- Preheat oven for 350°F.
- Prep tomatoes by removing stems and any brown spots. Place in cake pan or baking dish and drizzle with 1 tablespoon olive oil. Put in oven and bake for 45 minutes.
- Transfer tomatoes to blender and blend until very smooth. With the blender still spinning, add the rest of the olive oil, mustard powder, nutritional yeast, black salt, and calcium chloride.
- Pour mixture through strainer to remove any fibers or large un-blended pieces. Place mixture in fridge to cool and allow mixture to settle.
- Now, this part is tricky and may take practice. Have a bowl of cold clean water ready. Scoop out 1 tablespoon of the egg mixture and slowly drop into the middle of your alginate mixture. Trying to keep the blob of egg mixture circle-shaped. Using two spoons, one on each side of your tomato egg mixture, slowly push the alginate mixture toward the egg yolk in an upward motion. You are trying to cover and sink the yolk forming a sphere of skin over the yolk. The longer the yolk sits in the alginate, the thicker the skin. I only allow my yolk to sit for around 1 to 3 seconds. If you wait too long, then it won't be egg-yolk-like, and if you are too fast, the yolk skin will be too thin.
- Using a slotted spoon, slowly remove yolk from alginate and lower into cold water bath.
- Remove from water bath and enjoy.

Mung Bean Scramble Two Ways

Ever since I saw a company use mung bean protein to make an incredible vegan egg, I had to try to replicate it. My first version of this mung bean scramble actually looks more like a Korean mung bean pancake. I made it taste eggy, but it wouldn't really scramble; it always came out better as an omelet. Kind of a cake-like omelet but load it up with veggies and no one would know. For my second mung bean attempt, I took the process a little further. We are going to separate some proteins from their mung beans to make one of the most incredible vegan eggs!

INGREDIENTS

1 CUP SPLIT YELLOW MUNG BEANS

3 TEASPOONS BLACK SALT

1¼ CUP WATER

2 TABLESPOONS COCONUT CREAM

½ TEASPOON PAPRIKA

¼ TEASPOON TURMERIC

½ TEASPOON KONJAC GUM

DIRECTIONS

- Wash the mung beans well.
- Dry the beans first on a towel, then in a dehydrator at 140°F for 4 hours or until very dry.
- Blend beans into very fine powder.
- Sift through strainer, making sure there are no large grains left.
- Blend again to continue turning into powder. Should be finer than a fine flour, almost a starch consistency.
- Add very cold water to bean powder. Mix very well and let sit for at least 20 minutes. It can sit in refrigerator if house is warm. Keep it cool.
- Slowly pour mixture back into blender, watching for fibrous bits that have settled to the bottom of the bowl. Leave those behind.
- Add konjac gum, turmeric, paprika, coconut cream, and black salt to the blender and blend on a slow speed to mix.
- Heat a skillet on a low heat with a touch of non-stick spray or oil, cook until you see the top start to dry slightly, then begin to roll or scramble.

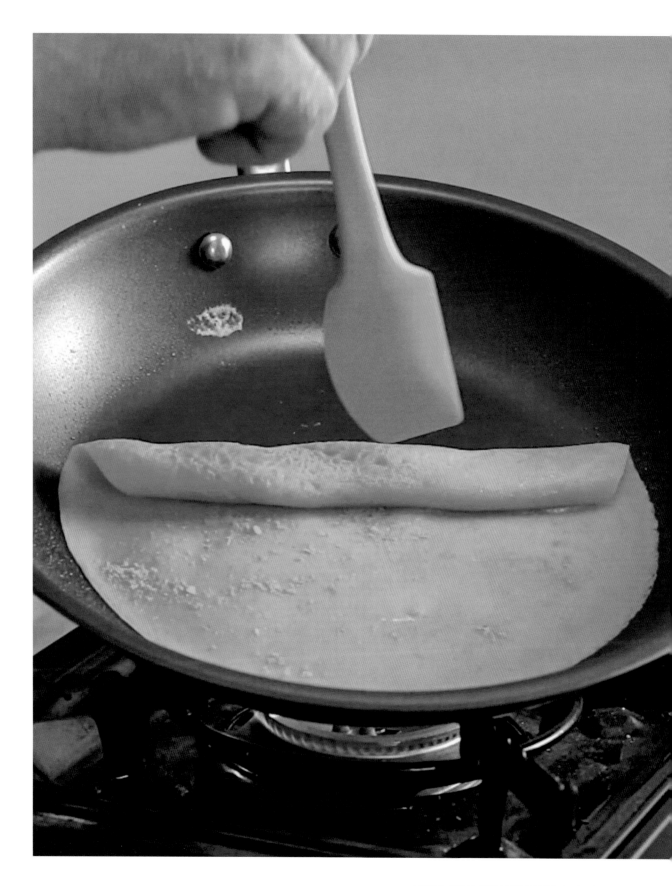

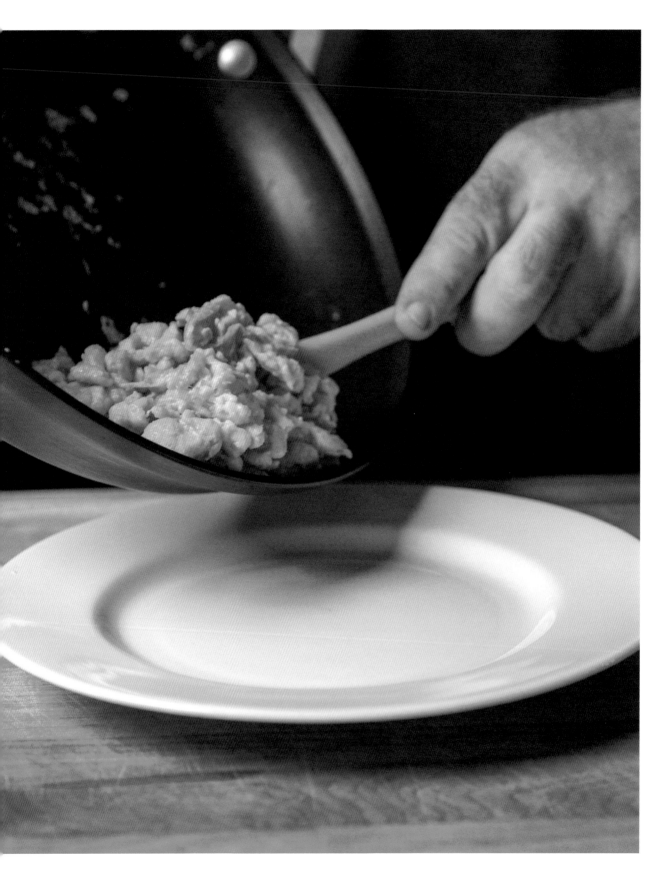

MUNG BEAN PROTEIN EGG

INGREDIENTS

1 CUP SPLIT HULLED MUNG BEANS
   OR MOONG DAHL

1 CUP COLD WATER

7½ CUPS COLD WATER

1 TEASPOON BAKING SODA

3 TABLESPOONS DISTILLED WHITE
   VINEGAR

2½ TABLESPOONS ALGAE OIL

½ TEASPOON ONION POWDER

½ TEASPOON TURMERIC

1 TEASPOON BLACK SALT (KALA
   NAMAK)

½ TEASPOON SUGAR

½ TEASPOON XANTHAN GUM

½ TEASPOON SOY LECITHIN

½ TEASPOON METHYLCELLULOSE

DIRECTIONS

- Start by blending mung bean and 1 cup of water to a butter-like consistency.
- Add baking soda to 7½ cups water, stir, then add to mung bean mixture.
- This mixture needs to be agitated for around 30 minutes. I recommend adding this to a stand mixer with whisk attachment, but this can be completed by hand.
- After agitating, slowly pour through nut milk bag. You will separate large fibers and starches here.
- Now heat the sifted water in a large saucepan until it reaches 84°F.
- Once the mung bean liquid reaches 84°F, slowly drizzle white vinegar into the liquid. You will immediately see the protein separating itself from the water! It's really fun to watch! Give this a very, very slow stir.
- Allow this to set overnight, covered and refrigerated. You will see the proteins settle to the bottom of the bowl.
- Using a turkey baster or siphon, slowly remove the liquid from the top of the protein. Try not to disturb the protein, as it will mix back into the water. You should end up with around 1½ cups of protein liquid.
- In a separate bowl, mix together the rest of the ingredients. This should get fairly gummy, then add the protein liquid and mix well!
- Now cook like a normal scramble in a nonstick skillet over a medium-low heat. Let cook for just a moment before you slowly start to scramble. This might take a little longer than a normal egg, but you should end up with a very light, fluffy scrambled egg.
- This can also be used as an egg replacer in most baking!!

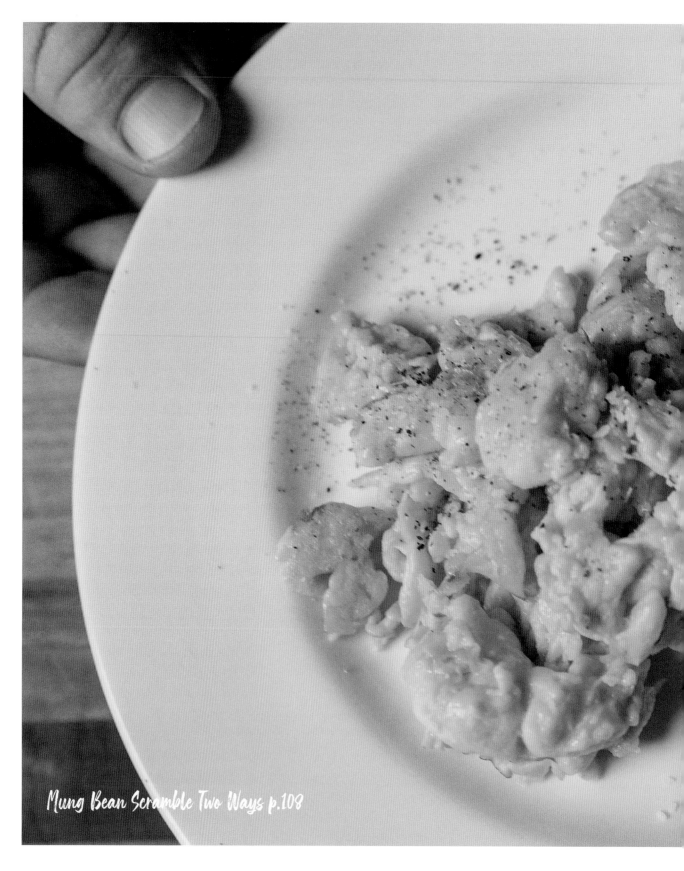

Mung Bean Scramble Two Ways p.108

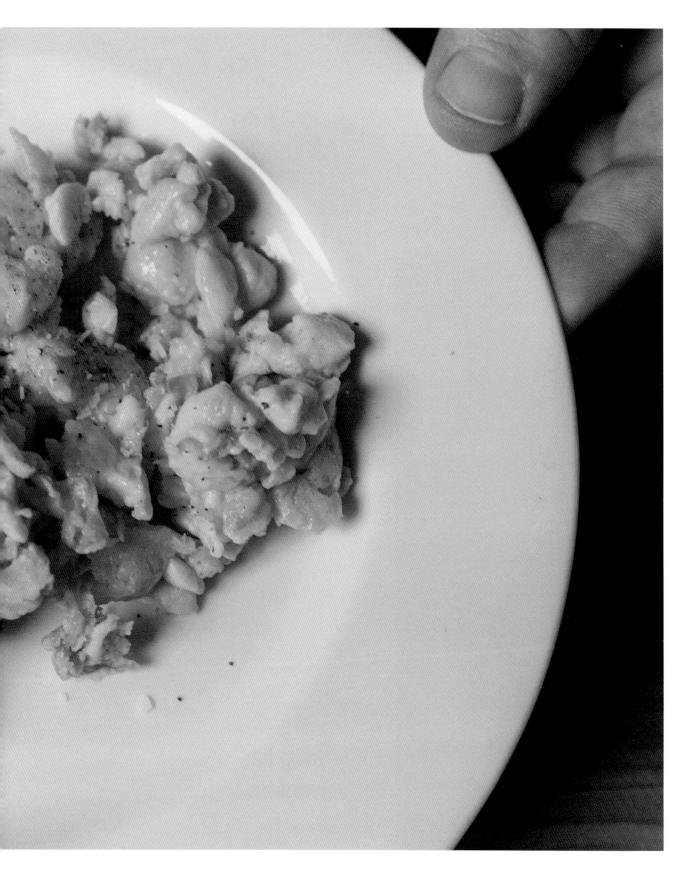

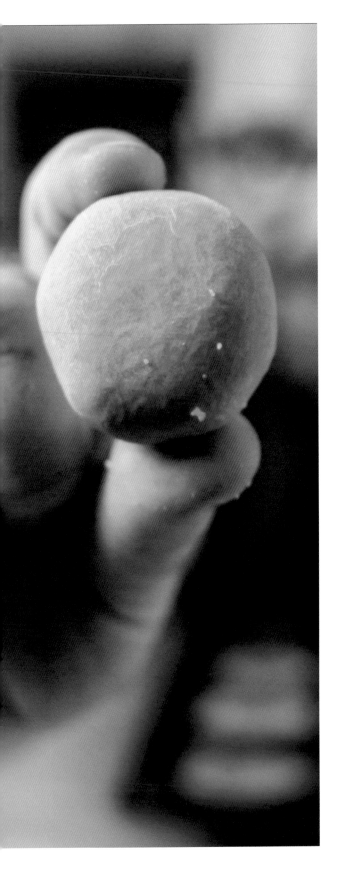

Vegan Cured Egg Yolks

When I first saw cured egg yolks I was blown away. You could take all the rich savory flavors of an egg yolk and cure it into a solid umami bomb. I needed to figure out a way to make it plant-based. It wasn't until I heard someone describe the cured egg yolk as being like cheese that a chord was struck with me on how to do this. Its texture was similar to a medium-hard cheese, and you could grate it and slice it. I knew what I had to do... Tapioca! One of my buddies (Not Another Cooking Show) makes these incredible Nutella tapioca balls. Essentially, they are Nutella mixed with tapioca starch until they are like a play dough. Now, tapioca when heated uncovered dries out fairly fast, and I knew I could make a cheese sauce that was flavored like an egg yolk from past recipes. So, once I combined everything together, we ended up with the first vegan cured egg yolk, and wow these things are good!

You can really use these "yolks" anywhere where you want added glutamate, added umami, super savory flavors! My easy go-to when I want an incredibly simple dish.

Cook up some bowtie pasta, drain, then coat with around a tablespoon or two of olive oil. Salt and pepper to taste, and make sure you use a flaky kosher salt for this. Top with some fresh basil, then, using a fine cheese grater or food planer, grate in almost half of one of these eggs.

You won't be disappointed!

INGREDIENTS

1 CUP CASHEWS

2 TABLESPOONS COCONUT OIL

1 TABLESPOON TOMATO PASTE

½ CUP COLD WATER

½ CUP NUTRITIONAL YEAST

2 TEASPOONS BLACK SALT

1 TEASPOON MUSHROOM POWDER

½ TEASPOON MUSTARD POWDER

½ TEASPOON TURMERIC

1 TEASPOON POWDERED AGAR AGAR

3 CUPS TAPIOCA STARCH OR
    TAPIOCA FLOUR

½ POUND OF KOSHER SALT

DIRECTIONS

- Cover cashews in boiling water and let set for 20 minutes to soften. Once soft, remove and rinse under cold water.
- Blend cashews with tomato paste, coconut oil, and water until smooth. Once you have a smooth consistency, add nutritional yeast, black salt, mushroom powder, mustard powder, and turmeric and blend to mix. Now add 1 teaspoon agar agar and blend one final time. The agar is added last to make sure the mixture doesn't heat and set prematurely.
- Now start adding tapioca starch, a half-cup at first, then a quarter-cup, until the mixture is a play dough consistency. This should take around 3 cups, depending on the humidity.
- Preheat oven to 250°F.
- Fill cupcake tray wells halfway with kosher salt. Press a round spoon or measuring spoon into the salt to make half-dome cups to set your "yolks" into.
- Now, using cold wet hands, roll the "egg yolk" dough into small balls, then slightly flatten to give them a yolk shape and place into the salt domes.
- Bake for 10 to 15 minutes or until yolk temp reaches 190°F (you will most likely have to sacrifice one yolk to get proper temp).
- Remove from oven and allow the yolk to come back to room temp, this should take around 20 to 30 minutes. Cover with more salt, then cover with plastic wrap.
- Place in the refrigerator and leave overnight.
- Next day, remove yolks and brush off salt! You can brush on more black salt if you would like, but these are ready to enjoy! Slice them or grate them into or onto your favorite soups, salads, sandwiches, burgers...I mean everywhere! These are *amazing*!!

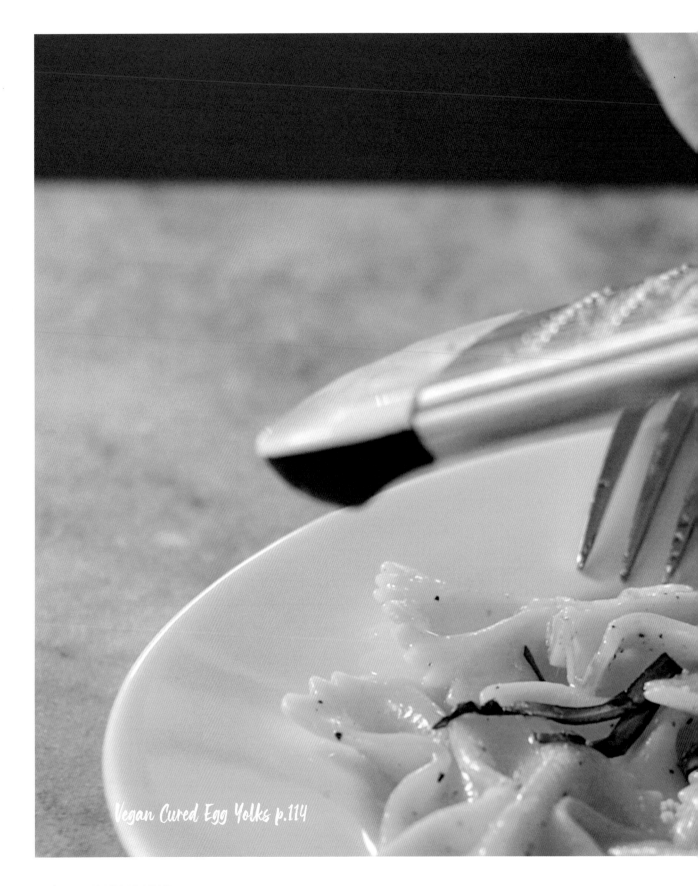

Vegan Cured Egg Yolks p.114

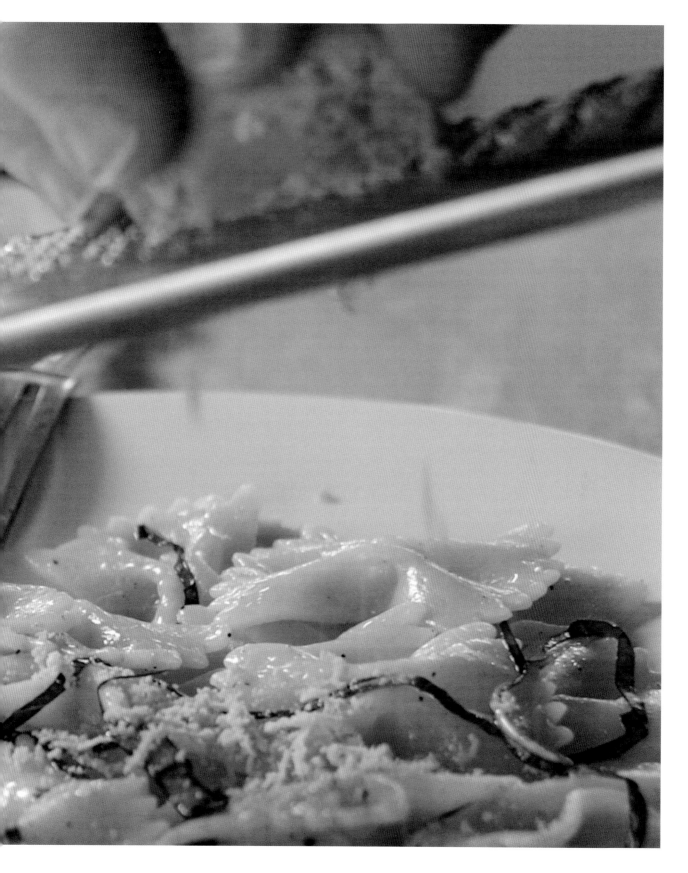

PORK

It's about time we took this book to the farm and saved our piggy friends. Most meat eaters I know always say they can't live without bacon. Well then, let me show you at least four bacon recipes to get that journey started for you, along with some pulled pork, a ham made out of a watermelon, and one of my favorite snacks to date!

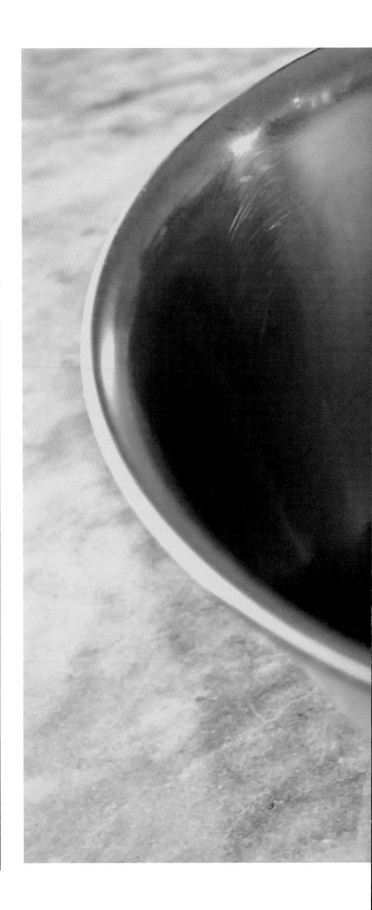

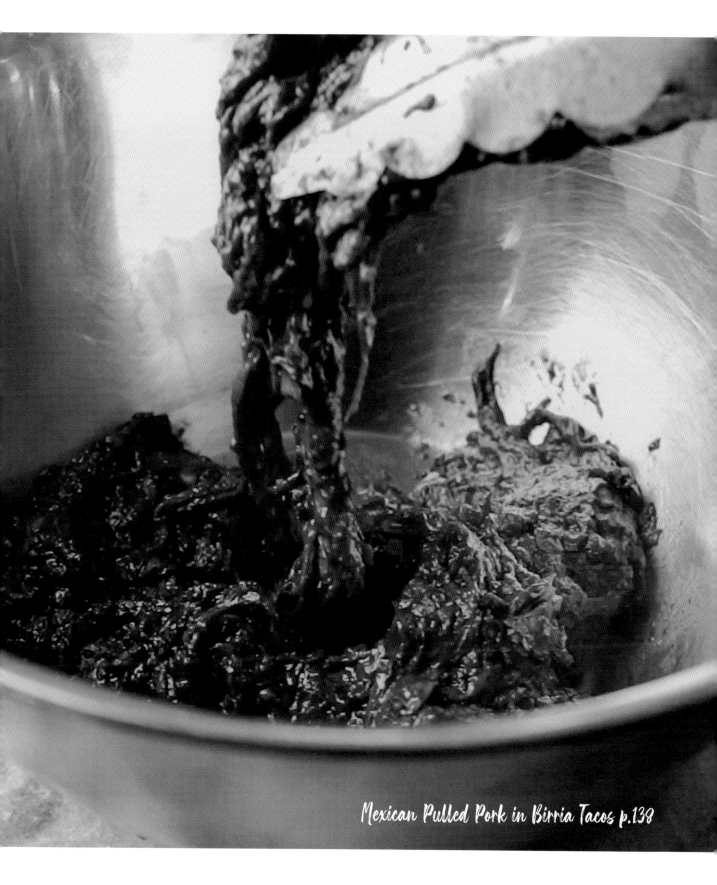

Mexican Pulled Pork in Birria Tacos p.138

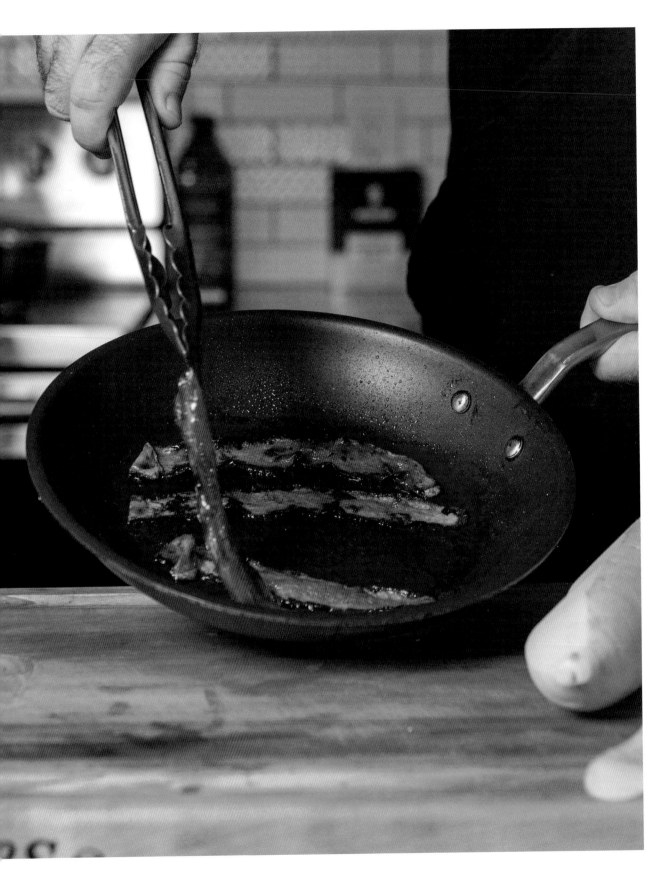

Daikon Bacon

I wanted to cover all my bases with plant-based bacon. Everyone has their own version of bacon they love, whether it's thick-cut bacon, thin bacon, crispy bacon, or soggy bacon. One of my favorite plant-based bacons is my favorite for a few reasons. It's easy, it crisps up pretty good, but it can also be a little soggy if you want it to be. I will always call this one, one of the tops, the daikon radish bacon.

This is the crispiest of the bacons in this book! And because of that I can wholeheartedly tell you to use this bacon in a...sandwich!

Grab two slices of your favorite bread, add some mayo to both sides, a little lettuce, tomatoes, salt and pepper, then load up that daikon bacon!

It really won't get much better than this.

INGREDIENTS

1 LARGE DAIKON RADISH
KOSHER SALT
⅓ CUP SOY SAUCE
2 TABLESPOONS OLIVE OIL
2 TABLESPOONS NUTRITIONAL YEAST
1 TEASPOON MUSHROOM POWDER OR MSG
1 TEASPOON LIQUID SMOKE
1 TABLESPOON MAPLE SYRUP
½ TEASPOON PAPRIKA
½ TEASPOON GARLIC POWDER
GROUND BLACK PEPPER TO TASTE

DIRECTIONS

- Clean the radish, removing the outside layer with a speed peeler.
- Using a peeler, press hard against the radish to create thick, wide bacon-sized strips.
- Lay the radish strips flat on a paper towel and cover with salt to pull moisture from the radish. Allow these to rest for 15 minutes while you mix your flavor marinade.
- Add the rest of the ingredients to a large bowl and mix well. Lightly add pepper, as radish already has peppery taste on its own!
- Clean the radish strips with a paper towel, then run under cold water to remove all salt!
- Place the strips into the marinade, making sure they are all covered, and allow to rest for 15 minutes.
- Heat a cast-iron skillet to a medium high heat and add about a tablespoon of oil.
- Fry strips in small batches, constantly turning so they don't burn. These burn really fast!
- Remove and allow to dry and crisp up on a paper towel or rack.

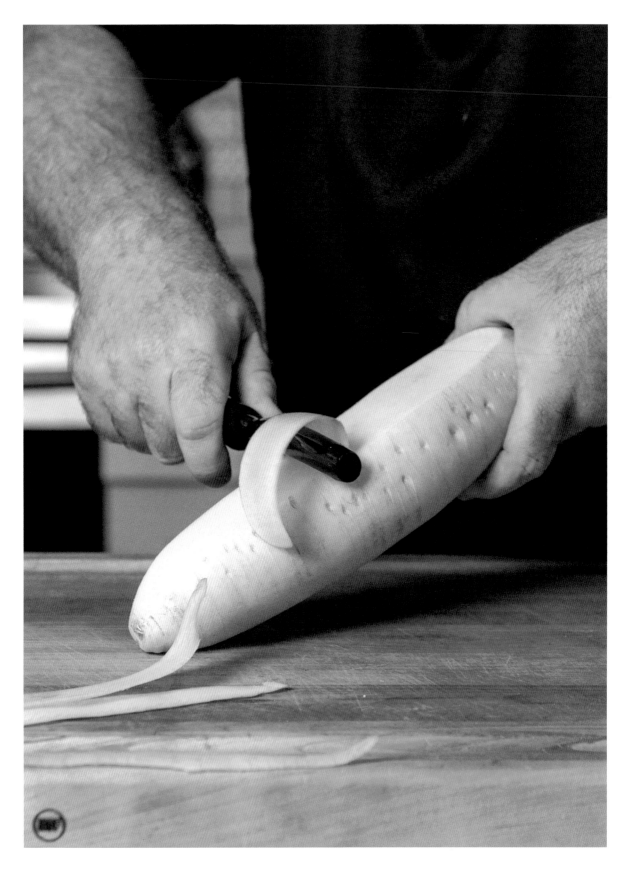

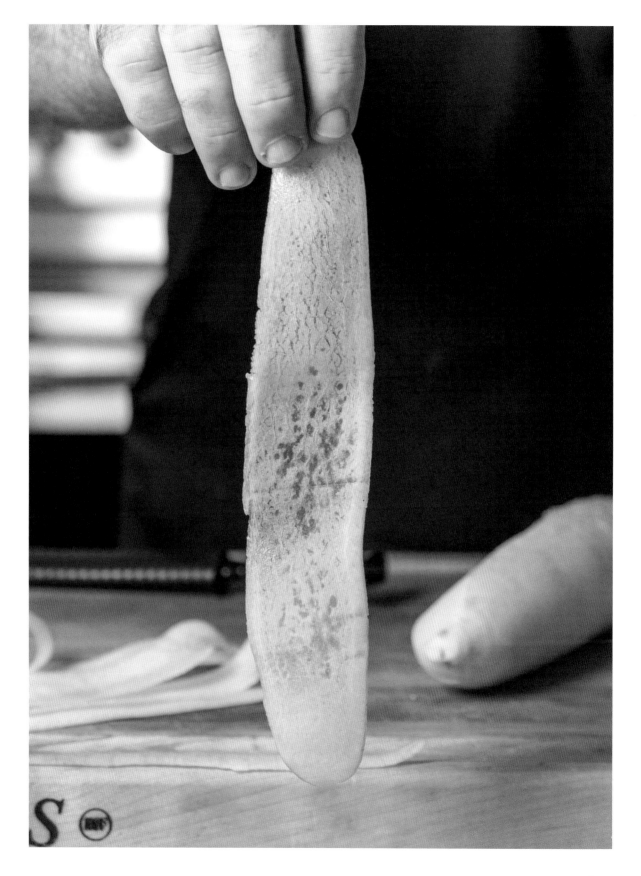

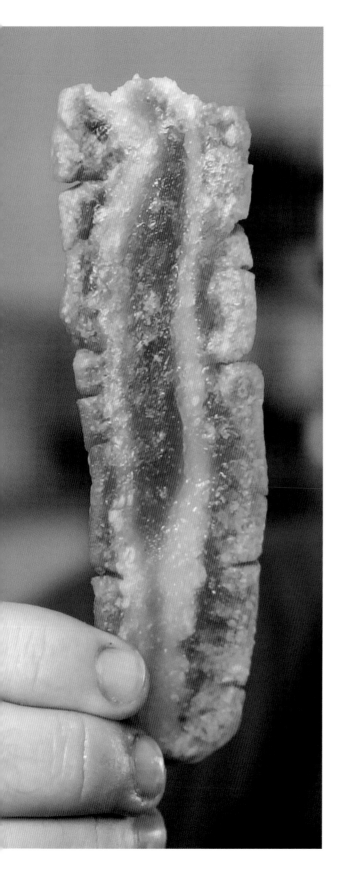

Thick-Cut Seitan Bacon

This bacon I discovered on Facebook, created by a gentleman named Nigel over at one of my favorite groups, the Seitan Appreciation Society. Nigel created a pretty epic bacon that I decided to tweak a little further to make my own. This is by far the king of plant-based bacon flavors and textures. Nigel wasn't the first person to make plant-based bacon using seitan, but he made it better, and that inspired me to use my knowledge of making bacon flavoring and nailing plant-based meat textures to step it up even one more notch. The fun thing about this bacon is that it can be flavored in so many different ways. Experiment with the seasonings that go into this to make a saltier version, maybe a sweeter version, or even a smokier version.

The seitan bacon is my favorite breakfast bacon. This works best when you pair it with one of the scrambles from earlier in the book! Little toast, mung bean scramble, and some fruit and you got a heck of a vegan breakfast platter!

INGREDIENTS

MEAT (RED PART)

1 CUP CHICKPEAS, LIQUID DRAINED
    AND SAVED (AQUAFABA)

½ CUP AQUAFABA (SAVED LIQUID
    FROM CHICKPEAS)

1 TEASPOON GARLIC POWDER

1½ TEASPOON SMOKED PAPRIKA

1 TABLESPOON MUSHROOM
    EXTRACT SEASONING

1 TABLESPOON SESAME OIL

1 TEASPOON MARMITE

½ TABLESPOON TOMATO PASTE

1½ TEASPOON LIQUID SMOKE

1 TEASPOON APPLE CIDER VINEGAR

½ TEASPOON MAPLE SYRUP

1 CUP OF VITAL WHEAT GLUTEN—
    DO NOT ADD THIS DURING
    PROCESSING STEP

FAT (WHITE PART)

½ CUP VITAL WHEAT GLUTEN

½ CUP AQUAFABA

DIRECTIONS

- First prepare the meat (red) part of the bacon by adding everything from the meat part into a blender or food processor and processing until very smooth.
- Pour blended mixture into bowl of stand mixer, or into another large bowl.
- Add vital wheat gluten to mixer and knead on a low speed until well combined, 5 to 10 minutes. You can do this step by hand simply by mixing the vital wheat gluten in with a large spatula or spoon, then kneading for 10 to 15 minutes on a gluten-floured table.
- Divide the meat dough ball in two and let rest while making fatty side.
- Now prepare the fat (white) part of the bacon. Add vital wheat gluten and aquafaba to stand mixer and allow to knead on low speed for 5 to 10 minutes, or mix in a large bowl, then knead for 10 to 15 minutes by hand.
- Now take the meat part and stretch into two even pieces that are as long as bacon, around 5–6 inches wide and less than a half-inch thick.
- Layer the fat white part on top of the meat part and stretch to cover. It's okay if this rips or tears, just make sure that you are covering most of the red part with the white part.
- Layer second meat part on top of white fat part.
- Then lay final fat piece on top of that and stretch to cover.
- Salt and pepper all sides.
- Wrap in plastic wrap and place in freezer until firm.
- Once firm, remove from freezer and wrap, and slice into very thin bacon slices.
- Fry on low heat with oil of choice, flipping once, until slightly brown and crispy.

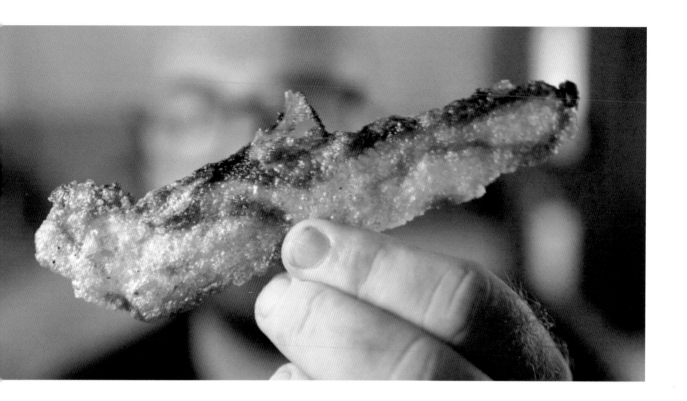

Bacon from Mochi (Sweet Rice Flour)

Now I want to take this bacon journey in a slightly off direction, an unexpected twist in the culinary plant-based meat road. I kept seeing this new vegan bacon popping up all over Instagram, and it looked incredibly real and I knew I had to figure out how it was made. I still have not figured out how that bacon was made, but during all the testing and screwing up, I did come up with my own version of that bacon: mochi bacon. This recipe is a testament to what testing and experimenting can create. I also recommend trying this particular vegan bacon sauce on some of my other vegan bacon recipes.

INGREDIENTS

RED INGREDIENTS

1 TABLESPOON MUSHROOM
    EXTRACT POWDER

2 TSP LIQUID SMOKE

1 TABLESPOON MAPLE SYRUP

1 TSP BEETROOT POWDER

1½ TABLESPOONS COCONUT OIL

2½ TABLESPOONS TAPIOCA STARCH

WHITE INGREDIENTS

1 CUP GLUTINOUS OR SWEET RICE
    FLOUR

1 CUP WATER

DIRECTIONS

- Combine all red ingredients together, whisk, cover and set in a refrigerator while preparing the next steps.
- Mix water and sweet rice flour together in a separate bowl. Whisk to combine.
- Cover and heat in a microwave on high power for 3½–4 minutes, stopping to stir every 30 seconds.
- Dust surface with rice flour. Remove rice flour dough from bowl and flatten using a rolling pin (cover rolling pin in starch or rice flour). You'll want the rice flour about a quarter-inch thick and as wide as strip of bacon.
- Cover the top of the dough ball with refrigerated red mixture. Using a spatula, make sure it's evenly spread over the entire top of the dough.
- Fold dough over onto itself and repeat until you have a thick piece of dough (half-brick size) with the white dough on the outside creating texture lines on the inside.
- Using a large square of parchment paper, tightly wrap the dough brick, then wrap it in foil to hold tight.
- Place in freezer until frozen solid, at least 2 to 3 hours.
- Once frozen, remove from freezer.
- Once the dough brick has thawed enough to slice, slice lengthwise into thin bacon strips.
- Heat a skillet on medium heat with a drop of olive oil and fry each slice until crisp, flipping only once.
- Remove from heat and place on paper towel or drying rack.

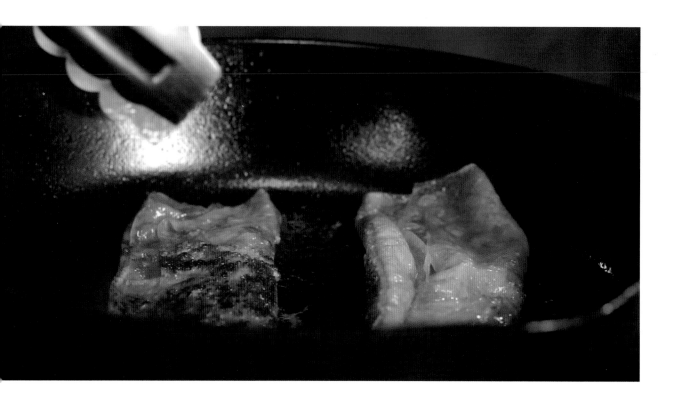

Soy Skin Bacon

Soy skin was one of my favorite go-tos when I first discovered it at my local Asian market. I was making it at home to wrap tofu or jackfruit chicken because of the way it crisped up to make a perfect meat skin. It was just such a simple transition to see if soy skin bacon would work. I quickly grabbed a piece of soy skin, cut it into bacon strips, flavored it, fried it, and wow, was I shocked. This one always ranks really high for me because of how incredibly simple it is. It doesn't tend to look like bacon, but if you like your bacon not crispy, then this is the one for you.

The soy skin bacon is such a great bacon to top off your favorite burger. It gets a little crispy, while staying chewy enough to top any of the burgers earlier in the book!! Top this on my TVP burger and you will have a burger win.

INGREDIENTS

4 CUPS ORGANIC SOY MILK

⅓ CUP SOY SAUCE

2 TABLESPOONS OLIVE OIL

2 TABLESPOONS NUTRITIONAL YEAST

1 TABLESPOON LIQUID SMOKE

1 TABLESPOON MAPLE SYRUP

¼ TEASPOON PAPRIKA

1 TEASPOON MUSHROOM SEASONING

½ TEASPOON GARLIC POWDER

GROUND BLACK PEPPER TO TASTE

DIRECTIONS

- To make the soy skin, we need to fill a 10- to 12-inch skillet with soy milk most of the way, or about 2 inches deep, and place on a medium heat.

- Once the mixture starts to heat, you will see a skin starting to form over the top of the soy milk. Allow this to develop into a thick skin that is covering the entire top of the soy milk.

- Using two spatulas, work around the edge of the skin to loosen it from the pan, then lift it gently from both sides out of the pan. This stuff is sticky when it's wet, so if it folds onto itself, it'll stay folded. Try to get pieces as large as possible. This takes practice!

- Place the soy skin over a rack to dry or hang over the edge of a large bowl, allowing the skin to drip. Do not let it dry to the bowl or it will stick.

- Once you have all your soy skin made, fold it into bacon-sized strips.

- Mix the remaining ingredients in a large bowl to make a bacon-flavored marinade, then place the soy skin into the bowl and allow to rest together for a moment.

- Heat a skillet over medium high heat with a tablespoon of olive oil and fry your soy skin bacon.

- Make sure to constantly turn so you don't burn the soy skin. Once desired color is reached, place on paper towel or wire rack to cool and crisp.

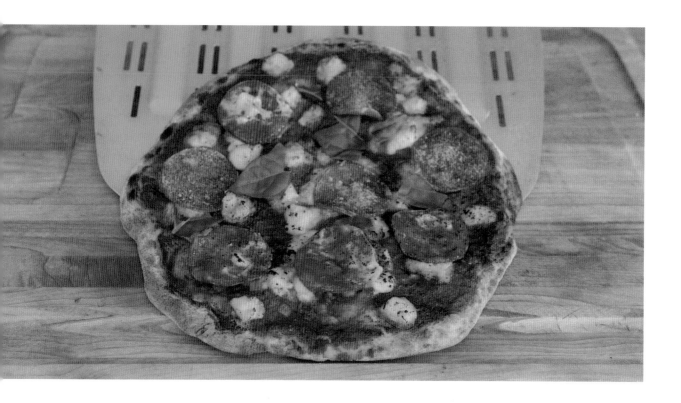

Wheat Starch Bacon and Pepperoni

Wheat starch is a fun starch to mess around with! There are a lot of things you can do with it as a binder, or a base for meats, but you can also make easy, simple vegan cheeses out of wheat starch.

I first started messing around with wheat starch after working with washed flour meat. That cloudy liquid you get when washing a ball of dough to make seitan is wheat starch. You can let that cloudy water rest and all the starch will settle to the bottom of the bowl. Once the starch has settled, you can pour off most of the water. What you want to keep is around a 50-50 mix of starch and water, almost the constancy of pancake batter.

For the next two recipes, you can use that pancake batter in place of the starch and water combination. You should have enough starch left from a ball of dough to fill around a half-cup. If not, add enough corn starch or water to the mixture to get to that half-cup of liquid.

WHEAT STARCH BACON

INGREDIENTS

RED "MEAT" BOWL

¼ CUP WHEAT STARCH

1 TABLESPOON TAPIOCA STARCH

1 TABLESPOON MUSHROOM
    SEASONING

1 TEASPOON SMOKED PAPRIKA

1 TEASPOON SOY SAUCE

¼ TEASPOON LIQUID SMOKE

1 TEASPOON MAPLE SYRUP

¼ CUP COLD WATER

WHITE "FAT" BOWL

¼ CUP WHEAT STARCH

¼ CUP COLD WATER

1 TABLESPOON MUSHROOM
    SEASONING

FOR COOKING

COOKING OIL

WATER FOR STEAMING

FLAT-BOTTOM CAKE PAN

LARGE SKILLET OR SAUCEPAN WITH
    LID THAT CAKE PAN CAN FIT INTO

LARGE BOWL FILLED WITH ICE
    WATER. LARGE ENOUGH TO SET
    CAKE PAN INTO

DIRECTIONS

- Mix all ingredients into their respective bowls.
- Add about 1 to 2 inches of water into your large skillet or saucepan and bring to a boil.
- Add a teaspoon of oil into the cake pan and wipe with a paper towel to spread a thin, even layer.
- Whisk your starch mixture right before you are ready to pour, as the starch settles quickly.
- Pour a thin layer of your red meat starch into the cake pan. Tilt and turn the pan to evenly distribute the mixture.
- Now pour thin lines of your white fat starch mixture and use a spatula to make steaky lines though the red starch.
- Lower the heat on the boiling water to medium, set the cake pan in the boiling water, then cover with lid.
- Cook for 3 to 4 minutes, then remove cake pan and set into ice bath. Be careful not to get the "bacon" wet.
- Once cooled, remove from cake pan. Slice into bacon slices, then fry in a skillet with a teaspoon of olive oil over a medium high heat.
- Remove to rack to dry and crisp.

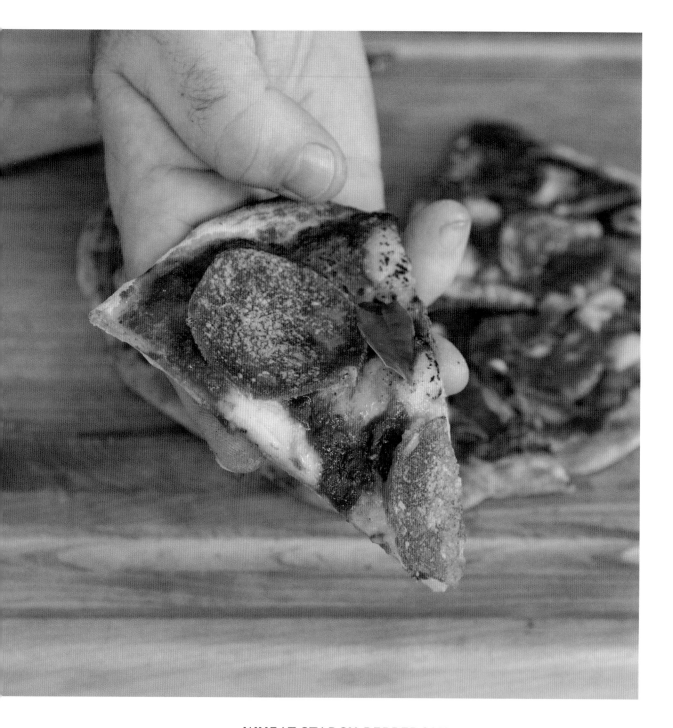

WHEAT STARCH PEPPERONI

The pepperoni version of this recipe has a few more steps! It's fairly simple, but *wow*, does it come out amazing! The great thing about this recipe is that, if you get your pepperoni thin enough, the pepperoni will actually cup up when cooking, just like real pepperoni! How wild is that?!

INGREDIENTS

RED "MEAT" BOWL

¼ CUP WHEAT STARCH

1 TABLESPOON TAPIOCA STARCH

¼ CUP COLD WATER

PEPPERONI SEASONING

1 TABLESPOON MUSHROOM
    SEASONING

1 TEASPOON SMOKED PAPRIKA

½ TEASPOON FENNEL SEEDS

¼ TEASPOON ANISE SEEDS

¼ TEASPOON GARLIC POWDER

PINCH CHILI POWDER

¼ TEASPOON SUGAR

¼ TEASPOON KOSHER SALT

WHITE "FAT" BOWL

¼ CUP WHEAT STARCH

1 TEASPOON KAPPA CARRAGEENAN
    OR 1 TEASPOON AGAR AGAR
    POWDER (OPTIONAL, THIS WILL
    MAKE THE FAT FIRMER AND
    CREATE A BETTER TEXTURE)

½ TEASPOON OLIVE OIL

¼ CUP COLD WATER

1 ADDITIONAL TEASPOON TAPIOCA
    STARCH, NOT TO BE INCLUDED
    IN INITIAL MIX

COOKING OIL

WATER FOR STEAMING

FLAT-BOTTOM CAKE PAN

LARGE SKILLET OR SAUCEPAN WITH
    LID THAT CAKE PAN CAN FIT INTO

LARGE BOWL FILLED WITH ICE
    WATER, LARGE ENOUGH TO SET
    CAKE PAN INTO

DIRECTIONS

- Mix all ingredients into their respective bowls. Put about 1 to 2 inches of water into your large skillet or saucepan and bring to a boil.
- Add a teaspoon of oil into the cake pan and wipe with a paper towel to spread a thin, even layer. Whisk your starch mixture right before you are ready to pour, as the starch settles quickly.
- Pour a thin layer of your white fat starch into the cake pan. Tilt and turn the pan to evenly distribute.
- Lower the heat on the boiling water to a medium heat, set the cake pan in the boiling water, then cover with lid. Cook for 3 to 4 minutes, then remove cake pan and set into ice bath. Be careful not to get the "fat" wet.
- Once cooled, remove from cake pan, roll into cigar shape, then slice into thin noodles. Then roughly chop the thin noodles into small chunks. Put the small chunks into a bowl, then add tapioca starch and mix to cover.
- Put your seasonings into a mortar and pestle or a grinder (even a blender) and crush or blend until seeds are well crushed and mixed. Mix this into your "meat" bowl starch. It should start to smell a lot like pepperoni and be fairly pink-colored.
- Add about half of the fat chunks to your meat mixture and whisk together. Now repeat the cooking process you did with the fat. You should be able to get two. Now that your large pepperoni slice is cooked, remove it from the pan and brush both sides with tapioca starch and melted coconut oil.
- Set the large pepperoni into the freezer for the coconut oil to set firm. Once firm, cut into small pepperoni shapes using a small cookie cutter. I just used the lid from a seasoning jar! You can now top all the pizzas you want!

Famous Smoked Watermelon Ham

Our next recipe was again inspired by Ducks Eatery. This one was viral, the world-famous watermelon ham. When I first tackled breaking down what the process could possibly be, I had to really dive deep into what brining techniques are commonly used and what flavors are most prominent in smoked ham. Lots of salt, sugar, seasonings. I didn't have to worry about the sugar, since the watermelon naturally had that covered, so for the most part, I just needed to add some glutamates through soy sauce and the rest of a standard brine. I have to admit that this one is a *lot* of work, but worth it in the end. It won't taste like ham, but it definitely tastes good and is wild to bring to a party.

You'll want to top this with something that's really rich, and I recommend a gravy. You can make a simple smoky, meaty gravy by using the drippings from the watermelon ham! Once the watermelon ham is cooked, remove it from the skillet and make sure you still have a decent amount of "juice" from the ham. At least a tablespoon worth.

Add 1 tablespoon vegan butter to the pan and melt, whisking around, gathering up any pieces left on the bottom of the skillet, then slowly add all-purpose flour about 1 tablespoon at a time until you get a smooth paste. About a half-cup or less of flour should do the trick. Add 4 cups unflavored soy milk or pea protein milk and whisk over a medium heat until it's a thick gravy consistency. Salt and pepper to taste!

INGREDIENTS

YOU WILL NEED A SMOKER!

1 LARGE "PEELED" WATERMELON

BRINE

1 CUP KOSHER SALT

1 TABLESPOON OREGANO

2 TABLESPOON CORIANDER

FRESH SPRIG OF OREGANO

1 TABLESPOON OAK WOOD ASH

1 CUP SOY SAUCE

2 CUPS HOT WATER

DIRECTIONS

- In a large bowl, mix hot water and all brine ingredients until salt is dissolved.
- In a bucket or ice chest large enough to fit the watermelon, fill around halfway with ice and water and your brine mixture. Drop the watermelon in the bucket and add more water if needed. Brine the watermelon for 48 hours. Check the temp, keeping it at 40°F by adding more ice as needed.
- After two days, remove watermelon from brine and place on baking sheet or sheet pan that will fit in your smoker. Smoke over indirect heat for around 8 hours. I used an apple wood for the smoke. Smoke until you have a nice leathery skin on the outside and the watermelon has reduced in size.
- Remove from smoker and save any liquid in the sheet pan. Do a cross-score across the top of the watermelon around 1 inch deep.
- Heat an iron skillet over medium heat with around a half-inch of olive oil and a few sprigs of rosemary. Carefully place the watermelon into the hot oil. I used two large spatulas.
- Using a spoon, baste the watermelon with the oil and sauté the watermelon uncovered for 15 minutes in the oil, constantly basting.
- Remove from the skillet to a large cutting board. Let rest for just a few moments, then slice.

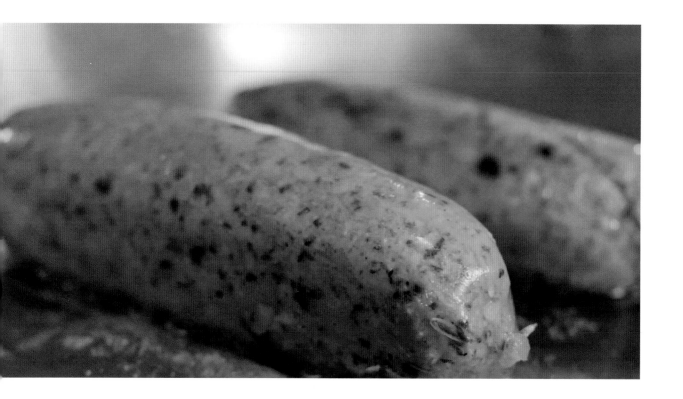

Beyond Good Sausage

Where I grew up, everyone loved sausage. There are so many different kinds of sausage, from Italian sausage to breakfast sausage, spicy or mild, but it all starts from the same base. That is what I wanted to give you here. This sausage is beyond good, a little tricky to make but it'll come out just as good as anything you can buy in the store. The version I am sharing is an Italian sausage version, but with a few tweaks you can make it like a breakfast sausage or your favorite German sausage. If this were a painting, I'd be handing you the blank canvas.

The only way I eat the sausages I make here is with onions and peppers sautéed in vegan butter until translucent, then coated with a touch of tomato paste and a small pour of tomato sauce, just enough to cover the peppers and onions. Once you're done making the sausages, either in a skillet or on a grill, slice up and mix with pepper mixture and enjoy! Did you ever have sausage, onions, and peppers like this at a wedding? Or is that just an Ohio thing?

INGREDIENTS

FOR THE MEAT

1 CUP TVP

1 TABLESPOON PEA PROTEIN
    POWDER

1 CUP DISTILLED COLD WATER

1 TABLESPOON NUTRITIONAL YEAST

1 TEASPOON SALT

1 TEASPOON BLACK PEPPER

1 TEASPOON DRIED PARSLEY

1 TEASPOON DRIED BASIL

½ TEASPOON PAPRIKA

1 TEASPOON RED PEPPER FLAKES

½ TEASPOON FENNEL

1 TEASPOON BROWN SUGAR

1 TEASPOON GARLIC POWDER

1 TEASPOON ONION POWDER

⅛ TEASPOON DRIED OREGANO

⅛ TEASPOON DRIED THYME

1 TABLESPOON COCONUT OIL

1 TABLESPOON CANOLA OIL

1 TEASPOON SUNDRIED TOMATO OIL,
    FROM THE JAR

1 TEASPOON MARMITE OR SOY
    SAUCE

½ TEASPOON LIQUID SMOKE

1 TEASPOON METHYLCELLULOSE

½ TEASPOON KONJAC FLOUR

FOR THE CASING

2 CUPS DISTILLED WATER

5 TEASPOONS SODIUM ALGINATE

½ CUP DISTILLED WATER

1 TEASPOON CALCIUM CHLORIDE

DIRECTIONS

- First, make the casing mix. To do this, you will need a blender. Mix the sodium alginate with 2 cups of distilled water. This needs to be distilled to make sure the sodium doesn't react to any calcium in the water. Pour this mixture into a tall cup and let rest refrigerated overnight or for a few hours, for the bubbles to settle. You can distinctly see the bubbles.

- The next day, combine 1 cup of cold water, TVP, and pea protein. Mix well and let rest refrigerated for at least 30 minutes.

- Put the TVP mixture into a large bowl along with everything else for the meat. Do not add the casing ingredients. Mix together very well and let rest for 20 minutes.

- Using square sheets of plastic wrap, form the meat mixture into sausage shapes, then roll the plastic wrap around the meat mixture. Twist the ends, then place in freezer to freeze.

- Once the meat has been frozen, mix the half-cup of distilled water and the calcium chloride in a spray bottle. (I've also done this by dipping, but I feel like the spray bottle works better. You can put the calcium mixture into a large cup for the next step.)

- Skewer the frozen sausage with a long skewer and dip sausage into alginate gel and wipe off excess, allowing a thin membrane to remain.

- Immediately spray sausage with calcium, then, after 30 seconds, dip into clean water bath (or dip briefly into calcium mixture, 5 seconds max).

- Cook sausage links in pan with a bit of oil, cooking to brown the meat or on a grill!

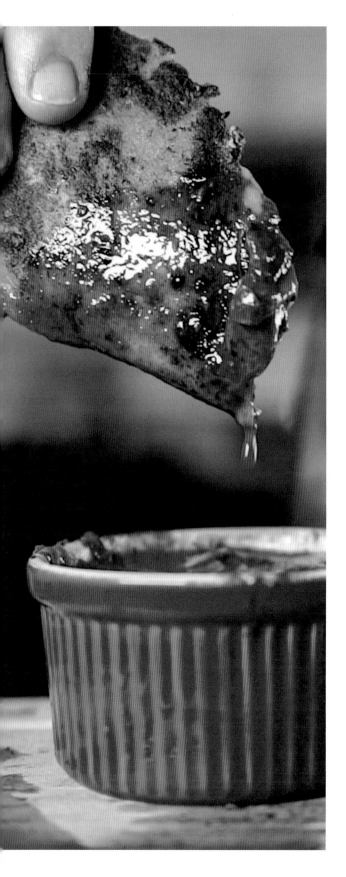

Mexican Pulled Pork in Birria Tacos

I have been seeing the messy, drippy tacos all over the internet. The birria taco and these tacos look insanely good. Tacos are by far one of my favorite things...so are rich meaty stews. So are messy foods. This is the combination of all of those. I did my research and put together what I felt would be a very viable vegan version of the birria taco. It might not be perfectly authentic, but it's incredibly good. If you can get your hands on these soy strands, the possibilities are endless for what you can do. Use them in place of TVP for any recipe listed here. For this recipe, it's fun to experiment with using young green jackfruit. It is easier to find, and you can quickly see how this amazing fruit can be turned into any "pulled meat."

INGREDIENTS

2 CUP SOY CURLS OR DELICIOU
   PLANT-BASED CHICKEN
   (YOU CAN ALSO USE CANNED
   JACKFRUIT)

3 CUPS WATER

1 TABLESPOON WHITE VINEGAR

1 TEASPOON MARMITE

1 TEASPOON SOY SAUCE

1 TABLESPOON OLIVE OIL

2 TABLESPOONS MUSHROOM
   SEASONING

10 ANCHO CHILIS

3 GUAJILLO CHILIS

½ YELLOW ONION, MINCED

½ HEAD OF GARLIC, MINCED

1 TABLESPOON OLIVE OIL

1 CAN FIRE-ROASTED DICED
   TOMATOES

4 CUPS WATER

1 TABLESPOON CUMIN

1 TABLESPOON OREGANO

1 TEASPOON SALT

5 BAY LEAVES

5 CLOVES

1 TEASPOON BLACK PEPPERCORN

1 CINNAMON STICK

VEGAN CHEESE

CILANTRO

DIRECTIONS

- Add your protein choice along with 3 cups water, vinegar, Marmite, soy sauce, olive oil, and mushroom seasoning to a large saucepan or skillet. Stir and cook on a medium heat.
- De-stem and de-seed chili peppers, add to protein mixture and allow to simmer covered for 20 minutes.
- Once the chilis are soft and have simmered with your protein, move the chilis to a blender along with a cup of the broth from the protein mixture and blend into a thick paste.
- Strain the protein and move to a lightly oiled Dutch oven or large saucepan to brown the meat over a medium high heat.
- Once the protein has browned, remove it and set aside. The bottom of the pan should be nicely coated with the browned seasoning.
- To prepare your consomé, add another tablespoon of olive oil to the pan and simmer your onions and garlic until translucent. Stir to coat with all the seasonings left from the protein.
- Add the canned tomatoes, the remaining liquid broth from the original protein mixture, and most of the chili paste (to taste). Add 4 cups of water to the onion mixture and stir to combine.
- Add the cumin, oregano, and salt.
- Now, using cheesecloth or clean cotton cloth, make a seasoning pouch with the bay leaves, cloves, peppercorn, and cinnamon. Wrap tightly and place over side of Dutch oven and cover with lid to hold in place. Simmer for 30 to 45 minutes.
- Prepare your fresh corn tortillas.
- Dunk tortillas into consomé, then cook in a lightly oiled skillet, cover with your vegan cheese, allowing it to melt a bit, then top with your protein, onions, and cilantro, fold over and cook both sides crispy.
- To plate, serve with a cup of consomé topped with minced red onion and cilantro.
- Dip tacos in consomé and enjoy.

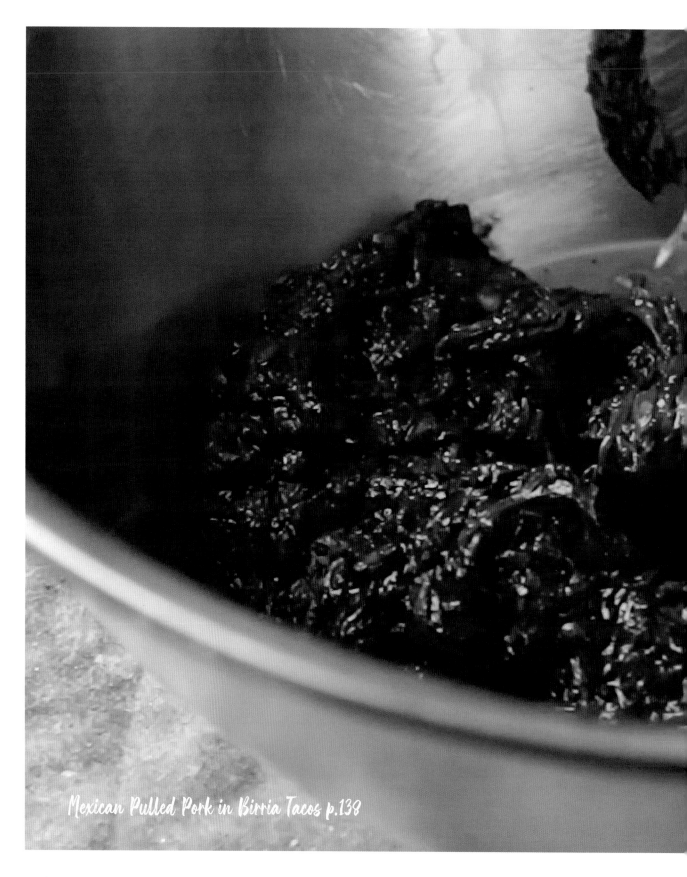

Mexican Pulled Pork in Birria Tacos p.138

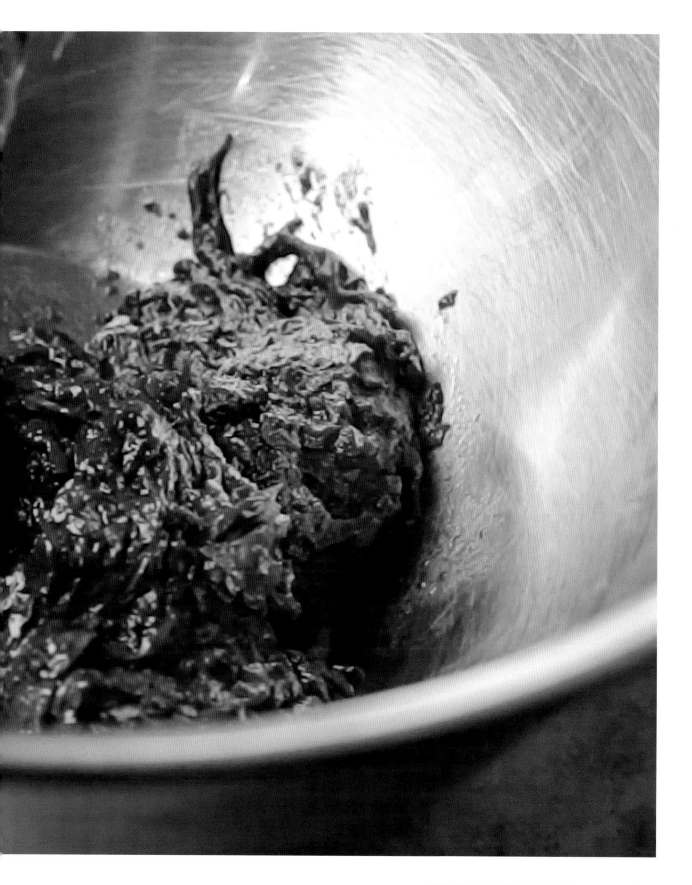

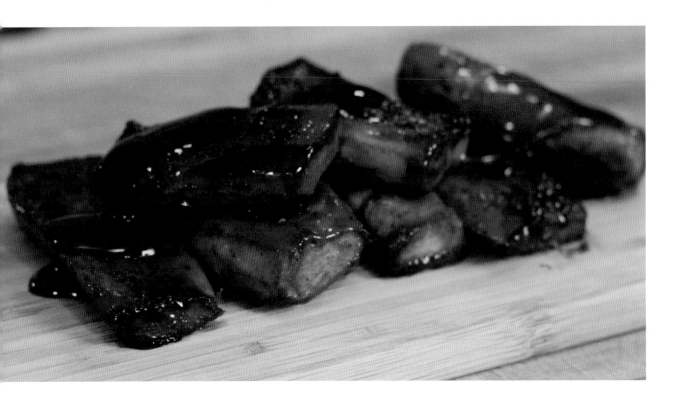

BBQ Mushroom Ribs

You can't talk about pork without talking about BBQ ribs. This is a recipe inspired by Derek Sarno. These are by far the closest and the only way I would recommend (at the time of writing this book) of making a vegan rib. They are juicy, have a nice bite and tear, and satisfy any BBQ rib craving or vegan curiosity someone might have. Even if you are not in the mood for ribs, these BBQ mushrooms are incredible. I love the versatility of the king oyster mushroom. Ribs, to back, to chicken...the king oyster can do just about anything meaty.

I don't know about you, but I feel like the only thing I want to eat BBQ mushroom ribs with is a summer macaroni salad.

Mix together

- 8 oz macaroni noodles, cooked
- ½ diced red pepper
- 2 stalks sliced celery
- ¼ diced red onion
- 1 cup vegan mayo
- 1 tablespoon apple cider vinegar
- 2 tablespoons pickle juice
- 2 tablespoons Dijon mustard
- ¼ teaspoon garlic powder
- ½ teaspoon paprika

Salt and pepper to taste

Then chill in the refrigerator for an hour or two while you make the ribs!

INGREDIENTS

6 KING OYSTER MUSHROOMS, MEDIUM-SIZE

1 TABLESPOON MUSHROOM EXTRACT SEASONING

1 TEASPOON SALT

1 TEASPOON CUMIN

1 TEASPOON GARLIC POWDER

1 TEASPOON CHILI POWDER

1 TEASPOON BLACK PEPPER

1 TEASPOON SMOKED PAPRIKA

½ TEASPOON DRY MUSTARD

1 TEASPOON LIQUID SMOKE

1 TABLESPOON SESAME OIL

2 CAST-IRON SKILLETS (ONE LARGE, ONE SMALLER)

DIRECTIONS

- Clean and trim mushrooms. I like to brush mushrooms clean and remove the very bottom.
- In a large bowl, mix seasonings, liquid smoke, and oils, then toss mushrooms in mixture until completely coated.
- Preheat oven to 350°F.
- Heat one large cast-iron skillet with a little olive oil over a medium high heat.
- Heat a second, smaller cast-iron skillet, making sure this skillet has a very clean bottom. I like to brush the bottom of this skillet with a touch of oil after it's been heated.
- Place the coated mushrooms in the large heated skillet and press firmly to flatten mushrooms and sear both sides evenly.
- Place flattened mushrooms on baking sheet or baking dish, coating both sides with BBQ sauce and bake for 45 minutes.

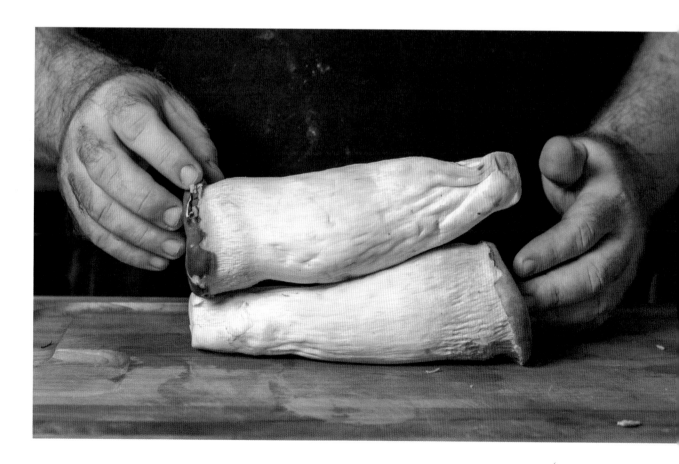

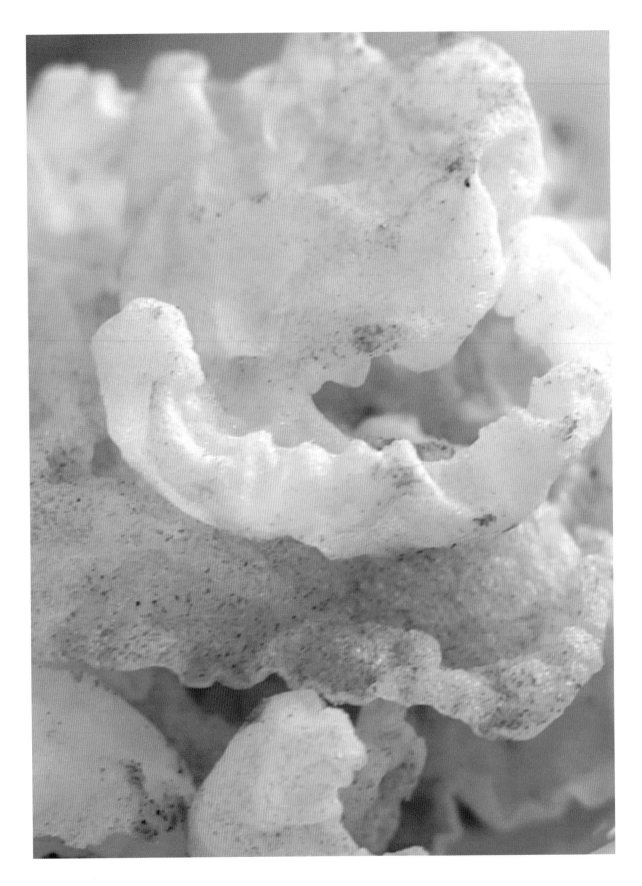

Porkless Pork Rinds

I always find accidental discoveries are the absolute best. They just feel so much more like an accomplishment. I discovered this one by accident for sure. I was wrapping a vegan chicken wing with rice paper and I wanted to see how it air-fried. After air-frying, the skin had bubbles on it and had a slight puff, so I immediately took a piece of dried rice paper, threw it in a skillet filled with hot oil, and *boom*, huge puff of rice paper. Now, after all that, I did a little Google searching and realized I wasn't the first to make puffed rice paper, but the accidental discovery still made this taste so much better to me... and to Monica. This is one of her favorite snacks.

INGREDIENTS

2 RICE PAPER SHEETS
COOKING OIL

DIRECTIONS

- Fill a large skillet with 1 inch of oil and heat to 375°F.
- Cut rice paper sheets into small rectangles, 1½ x 2 inches.
- Once oil is heated, drop 1–3 squares at a time. They will instantly puff up. As soon as they puff, remove from oil and allow puff to drip dry before placing in a large bowl.
- Season however you like!
- I like to season with a light drizzle of maple syrup, paprika, garlic powder, and a pinch of salt.
- You can try drizzling sesame oil, nutritional yeast, paprika, and salt.
- The flavoring combos are endless! Season as you would any popcorn or chip.

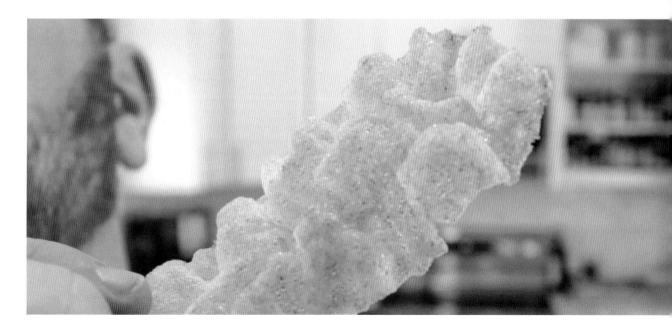

SEAFOOD

Now it's time we get off the farm and dive headfirst into the ocean with some seafood. I want to cover as many bases as I can, so you have a good start to making your plant-based seafood better. I am going to go over realistic shrimp, sashimi fish, and even a few fried fishes. We'll start with the easy ones and work our way up. All of these recipes can be tinkered with, explored, or taken apart to make something different, so feel free to give these a good mix-up!

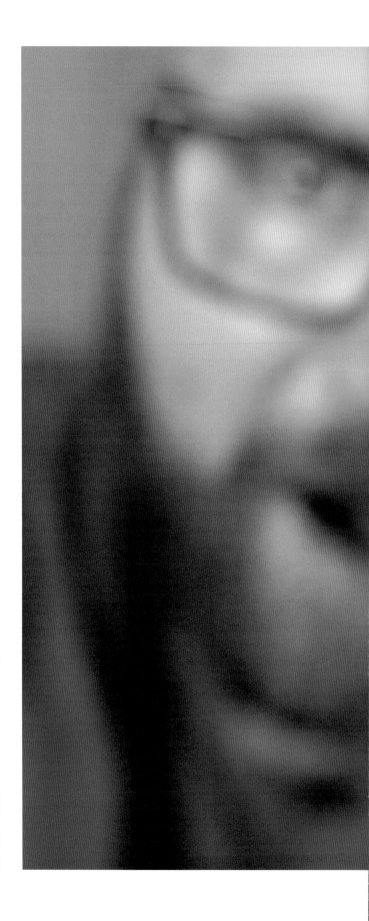

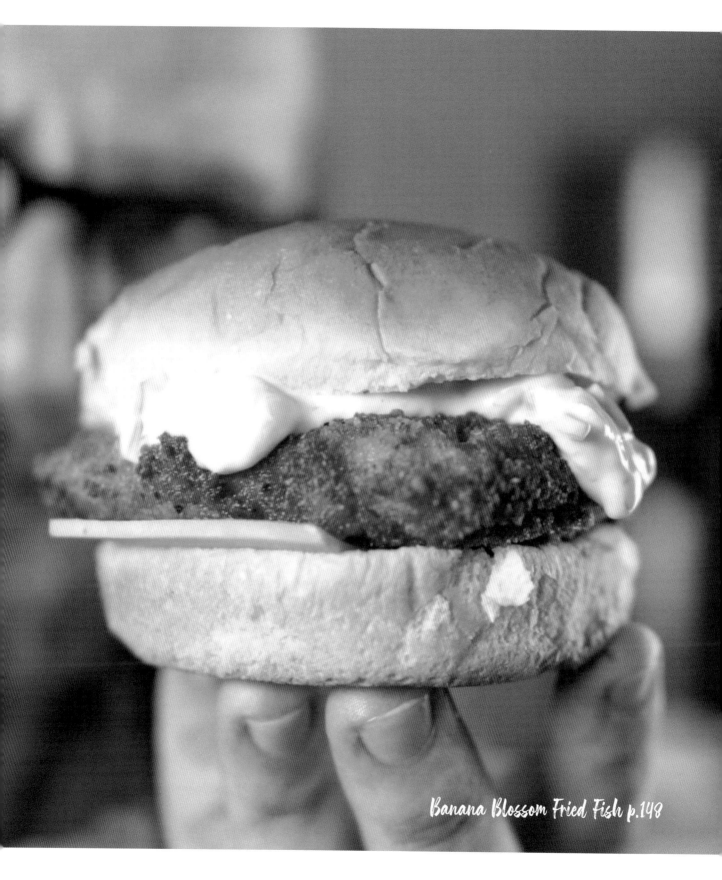

Banana Blossom Fried Fish p.148

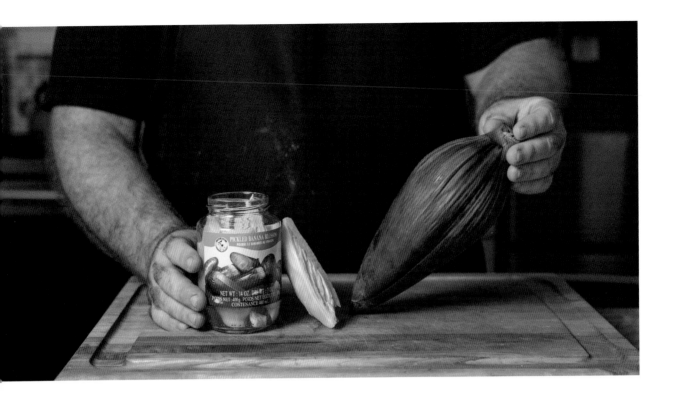

Banana Blossom Fried Fish

For this first plant-based fish, we are going to get you started the same way plants get started, with a blossom. This is the banana blossom fish. You can find canned banana blossoms at most Asian markets, and sometimes even at larger chain grocery stores. Sometimes you find them in the can in perfect condition and sometimes the layers are all torn apart. Either way, you will end up with a nice fishy fried fish that is just as flaky and delicious as its swimming counterpart.

Now, banana blossoms are also known as banana heart or banana flower. They contain some latex when you buy them fresh and require quite a bit of preparation before you get to the point where they resemble fish.

These fish fillets come out so tender and flaky, one of my favorite uses for them is in some Baja fish tacos! Throw the fried fish nuggets or fillets into a flour tortilla, then top of with one of my favorites.

Mix together

- 1 cup vegan mayo
- 2 teaspoons adobo sauce
- 2 teaspoons Sriracha sauce
- 1 teaspoon agave
- 1 teaspoon garlic powder
- 1 teaspoon salt
- ½ teaspoon pepper
- ½ teaspoon cumin
- ½ teaspoon cayenne pepper
- 1 tablespoon lime juice
- ¼ cup fresh chopped cilantro

INGREDIENTS

2 CANS BANANA BLOSSOMS IN
  BRINE, DRAINED AND RINSED

1 TABLESPOON KELP GRANULES

1½ CUPS FLOUR

½ CUP CORN STARCH

1 TEASPOON BAKING POWDER

20-OZ BOTTLE OF VERY COLD SODA
  WATER

1 LEMON

¼ TEASPOON TURMERIC

SALT

OIL FOR FRYING

DIRECTIONS

- In a large bowl, mix a half-cup flour, a pinch of salt, and kelp granules.
- In a second bowl, add 1 cup flour, corn starch, baking powder, turmeric, and salt. Mix to combine. Add the juice of a lemon, and slowly add soda water, whisking until the batter reaches a pancake batter consistency.
- Add oil to a large skillet, heat to 350°F.
- Roll banana blossoms in dry batter, then dip in wet batter and briefly into hot oil. Fry only a few pieces at a time, and don't over-fill your pan.
- Fry until golden brown. Remove to drying rack or paper towel. Salt to taste.

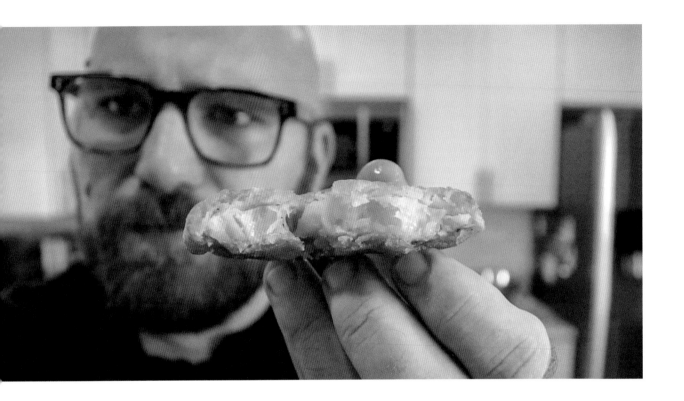

Celery Root Fried Fish

Celery is a unique thing in that it has almost no flavor yet loads of texture. Its cousin, the celery root or celeriac, is a unique root vegetable that has some of the same uniquely and faintly celery taste but with a really neat flaky texture, like it was crossed with a potato. With the right process of cooking and steaming, we can turn this weird root vegetable into a fish.

This is best made fried like I did here, but really the possibilities are endless. Wrap it in some seaweed or coat it with your favorite blackening seasoning and throw this in the oven for a baked fish. I would love to see how far you experiment with this one!

I say fish, you say tartar sauce. That doesn't really work, but tartar sauce goes hand in hand with fried fish, and it's easy to make!

Mix together, then let sit in the refrigerator for an hour!

- ¼ cup vegan mayo
- 2 tablespoons sweet relish
- 1 teaspoon minced yellow onion
- 1 teaspoon plant-based milk
- 1 teaspoon minced capers
- ½ teaspoon lemon juice
- ¼ teaspoon dried parsley
- 1 teaspoon agave

INGREDIENTS

3 CELERY ROOTS, PEELED AND
    CLEANED

2 TABLESPOONS OLIVE OIL

2 TEASPOONS SEA SALT

1 TABLESPOON KELP GRANULES

MARINADE

½ CUP OLIVE OIL

½ CUP RICE VINEGAR

1 TEASPOON CAPER BRINE

1 TABLESPOON CAPER

JUICE OF 1 LEMON

1 TABLESPOON SUGAR

BATTER

FLOUR, ABOUT 2 CUPS

1 TEASPOON BAKING SODA

1 TEASPOON SEA SALT

1 CAN CHEAP BEER

1 CUP CORN STARCH

VEGETABLE OIL FOR FRYING

DIRECTIONS

- Slice celery root into half-inch to three-quarter-inch-thick slices.
- Drizzle with olive oil, salt, and kelp granules, and toss to make sure everything is coated.
- Preheat oven to 400°F. Place celery root on a parchment-paper-lined baking sheet and pour remaining oil and seasonings over root. Roast for 30 minutes, then set aside.
- In a large bowl, mix together all the ingredients from marinade and put celery root into marinade, cover and refrigerate for 6 hours.
- In a large saucepan or Dutch oven, add about 3 inches of oil. Make sure you have a large enough pot. Never fill more than halfway up, for safety. Heat to 375°F.
- Mix batter ingredients together in one large bowl and corn starch in another bowl.
- Dip "fish" into corn starch to coat, then wet batter, then fry. Fry until golden brown and remove to wire rack. Do not overfill fryer, only do a few pieces at a time.
- Top with a pinch of salt and enjoy!

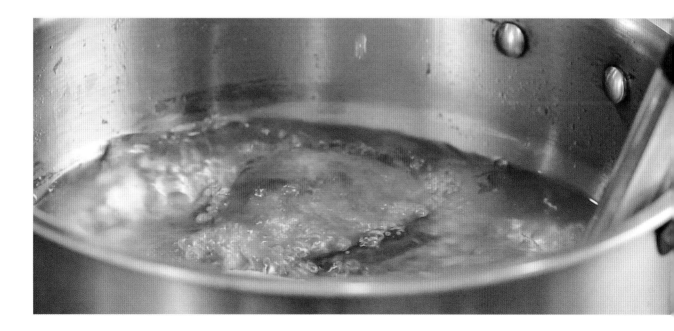

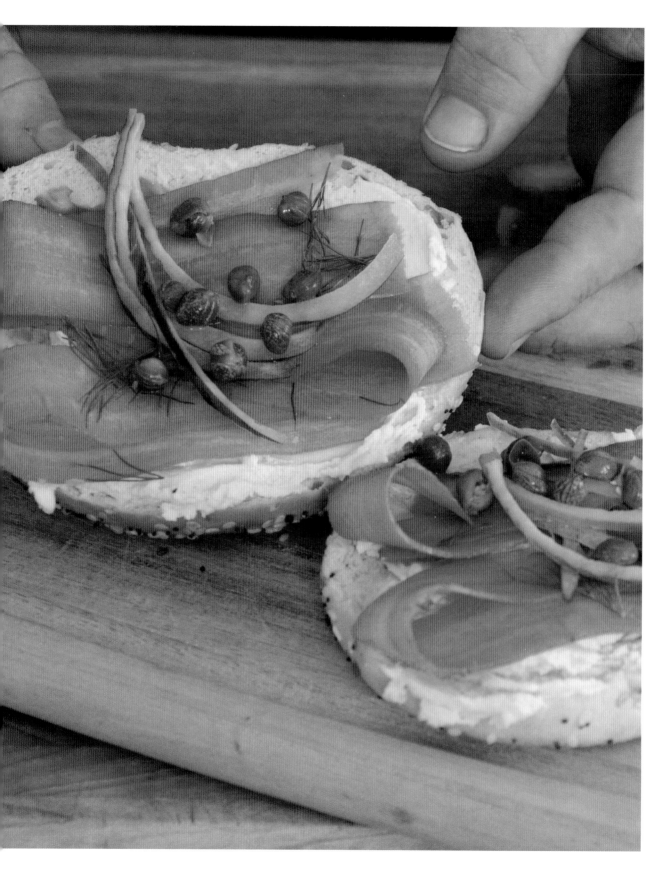

Carrot Salmon "Lox"

Lox and bagels are by far one of my favorite things, so when thinking about how to replace my fishy friends with some fishy plants, I didn't have to dive that deep. There are loads of ways to make a vegan lox that when topped just right you wouldn't even tell the difference… Gimme some capers and dill atop that lox and it'll be gone in a flash. This is one of the easiest of the seafood recipes, and can be used as you would use lox, but also in a quick pinch in place of salmon for sushi!

You can replace the carrots in this recipe with tomato skins, or even beets!

INGREDIENTS

3–4 CARROTS

2 POUNDS KOSHER SALT

1 CUP WATER

½ CUP SOY SAUCE

1 TEASPOON WHITE VINEGAR

1 TEASPOON CAPER BRINE

½ TEASPOON SMOKED PAPRIKA

¼ TEASPOON LIQUID SMOKE

½ TABLESPOON KELP GRANULES

1 TABLESPOON ALGAE OIL

DIRECTIONS

- Preheat oven to 425°F.
- Wash and clean your carrots, leaving wet. Use a baking dish, pour a bed of salt onto the baking dish, then place your veggies on the salt, then cover with more salt. Bake for 30 to 40 minutes.
- To a large bowl, add water and the rest of the ingredients.
- Once the carrots are done baking, allow them to cool completely and remove from the salt. Slice into thin slices and place in brine mixture. Cover and refrigerate overnight.
- Once done, remove from brine, top with capers and fresh dill, and enjoy!

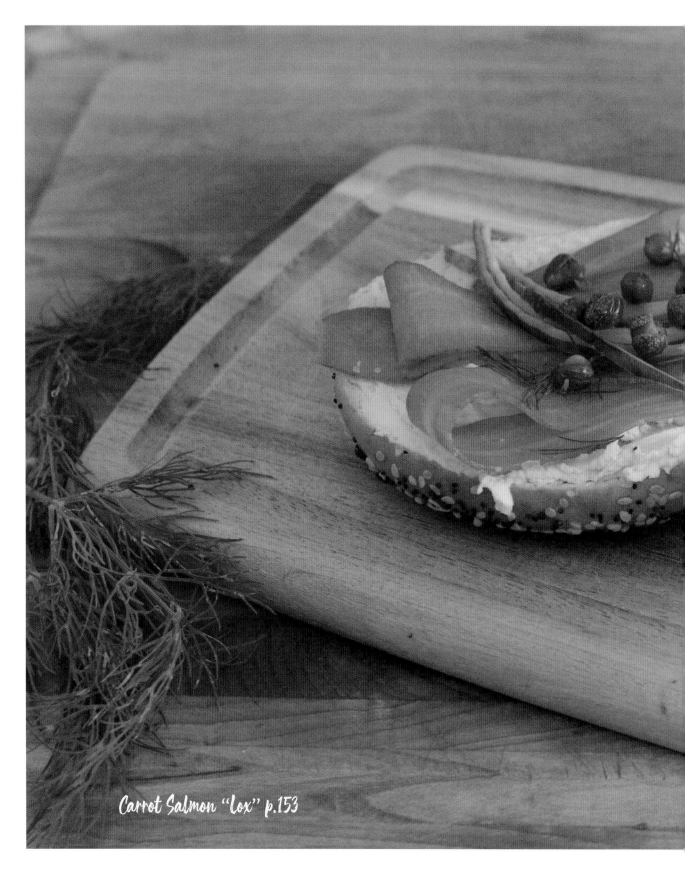

Carrot Salmon "Lox" p.153

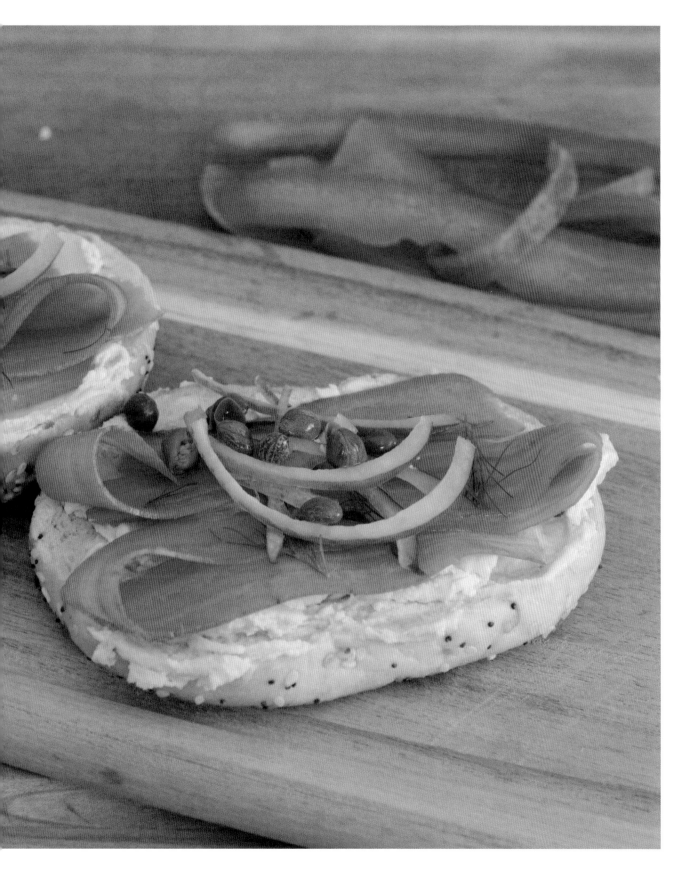

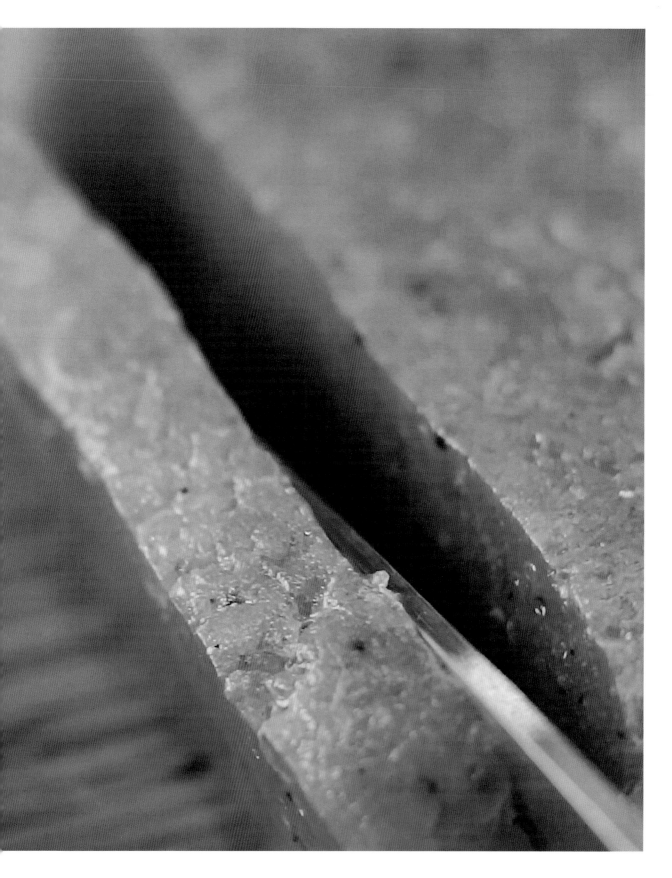

Vegan Sushi Fish

You've never had plant-based sashimi type fish like this next one before. This recipe came to me after trying a konjac cake from my local Asian market. These little square gelatinous cakes have the wildest fish-like consistency I've ever tried, and honestly even smell just like fish. I was absolutely shocked after making this one that this isn't used more widely in the plant-based seafood world. After seeing a few startups attempting to turn this ingredient into a viable seafood replacement, I knew I had to try my hand at it.

There are not many swappable ingredients in this one, besides the kelp powder. You can swap kelp powder for any seaweed powder, seaweed sheets, or sea-flavored seasonings.

You're obviously going to be making sushi or sushi bowls with this fish, right? Well, then you might want a simple sushi rice recipe!

- 2 cups rinsed and cooked short-grain rice—cook according to package directions
- 1 tablespoon salt
- ¼ cup sugar
- ¼ cup rice vinegar
- ¼ cup white wine vinegar

Make sure you rinse the rice clean before cooking. Why do so many of you skip this step?! It's a plant, wash it! And it's loaded with starches, which will gum up the rice and give it a not-so-nice texture!

While the rice is cooking, mix your salt, sugar, and vinegars in a small saucepan and heat over a low heat until sugar is dissolved.

Transfer your cooked rice to a large bowl, then slowly drizzle in the vinegar mixture and fold in. While folding rice mixture in, use a thin cutting board, piece of cardboard or piece of junk mail to fan off the rice. This will help dry the rice and give it its signature sticky texture!

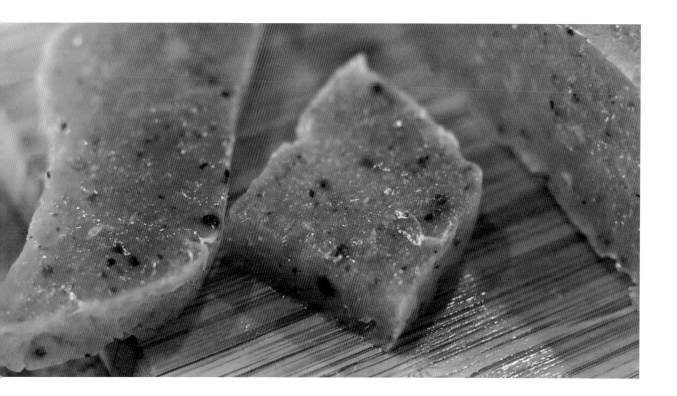

INGREDIENTS

2 TABLESPOONS KONJAC GUM

1 TEASPOON SODIUM ALGINATE

1 TEASPOON SEA SALT

½ TEASPOON KELP POWDER

½ TEASPOON PAPRIKA

3 CUPS WATER

ADDITIONAL 1 TABLESPOON WATER

1 TEASPOON AGAVE

1 TEASPOON OLIVE OIL

1 TEASPOON CALCIUM HYDROXIDE

DIRECTIONS

- In the bowl of a stand mixer with whisk attachment, or in a large bowl with a hand beater, mix together the konjac gum, sodium alginate, salt, kelp powder, and paprika until everything is distributed well.

- Heat 3 cups of water to 125°F, then add water to dry mixture while whisking on high. This will gel very rapidly.

- In a separate bowl, mix together water, agave, oil, and calcium hydroxide. Do not allow unmixed calcium hydroxide to touch skin.

- Quickly pour and knead mixture together with large wooden spoon, making sure that liquid is mixed throughout. This will have a rapid gelling effect. If you overmix, the texture will be brittle and loose. Mix only until incorporated. You will smell a fish-like smell.

- Quickly pour into mold and press. This can be a large bowl, bread pan, or small baking dish.

- Cover and let rest for 1 hour.

- After it's rested, boil in salted water for 30 minutes, then transfer to ice-cold water.

- Slice into thin slices for sushi, or cube for poke bowl, or dab on that wasabi and dip into soy sauce.

Lion's Mane Crab Cake

The lion's mane mushroom is one of my favorite mushrooms for a few reasons. It has an incredibly fun texture that is easy to work into a lot of foods, and it has a really mild crab-like taste. If you leave it alone and simply add it to other seafood-like flavors, you can really boost that crab flavor to make some incredible mushroom-based seafood dishes. This is a simple technique to make crab meat that can be used in any recipe where crab meat is needed.

When tossing with garlic and olive oil, add some kelp or seaweed seasonings to boost the seafood flavors!

You'll definitely want to top these off with a super simple, easy crab cake sauce.

- ¼ cup vegan mayo
- ½ teaspoon Dijon mustard
- ½ teaspoon paprika
- Juice of ½ lemon

Mix everything together, it's that easy.

INGREDIENTS

1–2 LARGE LION'S MANE MUSHROOM, AROUND 2 CUPS

3 CLOVES GARLIC, MINCED

2 TEASPOONS OLIVE OIL

1 EGG REPLACER, 3–4 TABLESPOONS LIQUID

1 TEASPOON SOY SAUCE

1 TEASPOON RICE VINEGAR

½ TEASPOON BLACKSTRAP MOLASSES

2 TABLESPOONS VEGAN MAYO

JUICE OF HALF A LEMON

1 TEASPOON DRIED PARSLEY

¼ CUP MINCED RED ONION

1 TEASPOON OLD BAY

¼ CUP PANKO BREADCRUMBS

½ CUP ITALIAN BREADCRUMBS

DIRECTIONS

- Shred lion's mane mushroom by hand. Toss with garlic and olive oil.
- Bake on a baking sheet at 350°F for 15 minutes.
- In a large bowl, add the rest of the ingredients and mix together well. Remove mushroom from oven when done and add directly to mixture.
- Form mixture into patties. Add water if needed to help stick.
- Salt and pepper to taste.
- Heat cast-iron skillet over a low-medium heat and coat with a touch of oil. Fry mushroom crab cakes until desired color.

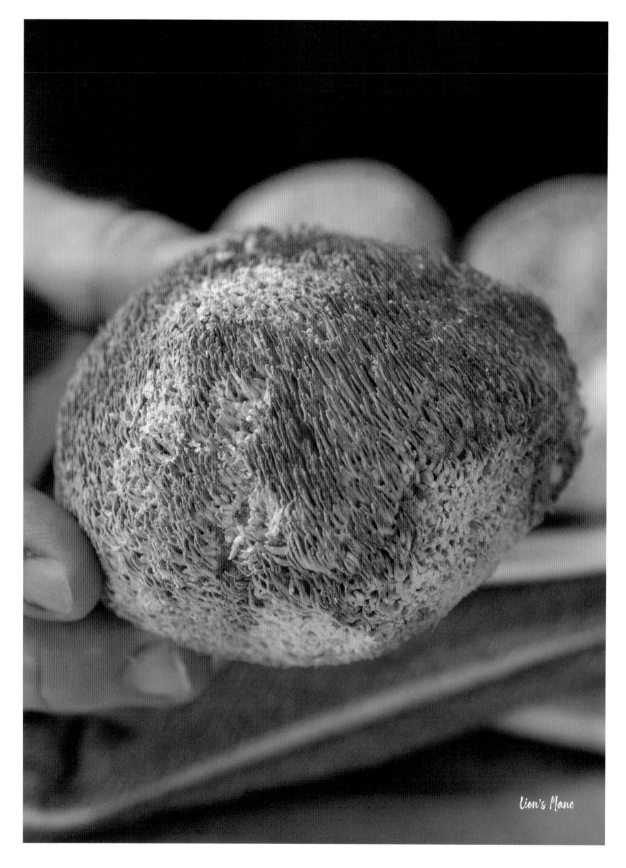

Lion's Mane

RESOURCES

YOUTUBE

The Edgy Veg:
Youtube.com/user/stillcurrentstudios

Thee Burger Dude:
Youtube.com/theeburgerdude

Mary's Test Kitchen:
Youtube.com/user/marystestkitchen

Gaz Oakley:
Youtube.com/avantgardevegan

Wicked Foods:
Youtube.com/channel/UCF4FF7ZzsDf-cxFg3g68eY5A

Modernist Pantry:
Youtube.com/c/KitchenAlchemyfromModernistPantry

FACEBOOK

The Seitan Appreciation Society:
Facebook.com/groups/MakingSeitan

The Washed Flour and Other Seitan Recipes and Methods:
Facebook.com/groups/1520295431471858/

ONLINE

Modernist Pantry:
modernistpantry.com

Vegan Gastronomy:
reefromthat.com

Google/Bing/DuckDuckGo:
Whatever it is you use to search on the internet, do some research. Look into what has been done to figure out what can be done. Nothing is impossible, and almost everything is figure-out-able.

INDEX

A
Agar agar: 17, 30, 46, 115, 133
Alginate: 18, 107, 137, 158
Arrowroot: 19, 85

B
Bacon: 13, 15, 18-19, 25, 28, 56, 86, 118, 121, 124-131
Banana blossom: 148
Bbq mushroom: 142
Bean curd: 24, 86-87
Beef: 16, 23, 25, 28, 30, 36, 40, 48, 59, 66, 68
Beet juice: 39-40, 46, 58
Beetroot: 24, 40-41, 46, 48, 53, 58, 63, 127
Beyond: 30
Birria tacos: 138
Black salt: 100, 103, 105, 107-108, 111, 115
Blackstrap molasses: 25, 39, 41, 45, 48, 53, 66, 159
Blender: 27, 31, 33, 39, 48, 53, 56, 85, 91, 105, 107-108, 125, 133, 137, 139
Brine: 16, 67, 134-135, 149, 151, 153
Burger: 22, 24, 28, 30, 38-41, 44, 48, 68-69, 128

C
Cauliflower: 87
Celery root: 150-151
Cheesecloth: 26, 33, 139
Chicken: 14, 16, 19, 25, 30, 40, 78, 80-82, 84-88, 90-93, 95-96, 98-100, 103, 128, 139, 142, 145
Chicken of the woods: 14
Chickpea: 39, 46, 48
Chickpea flour: 46, 48
Coconut: 24-25, 31, 48, 85, 93, 108, 115, 127, 133, 137
Coconut milk: 24
Coconut oil: 25, 31, 48, 85, 93, 115, 127, 133, 137
Crab cake: 159
Cured egg: 114

E
Egg: 18-19, 22, 24, 45, 57, 67, 69, 89, 91, 93, 95-96, 99-100, 102, 104-108, 111, 114-115, 159
Egg replacer: 19, 22, 24, 45, 57, 67, 69, 89, 91, 93, 95-96, 99, 111, 159
Egg yolk: 106-107, 114-115

F
Fat: 17-19, 25, 28, 30-31, 40-41, 48, 52, 69, 85, 125, 131, 133
Fish: 17, 56, 146, 148, 150-151, 157
Flour: 19, 39, 46, 48, 57, 62-63, 80, 82, 91, 93, 95-96, 99, 108, 115, 126-127, 130, 134, 137, 148-149, 151
Fried fish: 148, 150

G
Garlic: 39, 41, 45-46, 52, 56, 63, 67, 69, 74, 81, 89, 96, 99, 105, 121, 125, 129, 133, 137, 139, 142-143, 145, 148, 159
Glutamate: 25, 114
Gluten: 22, 36, 45, 48, 62-63, 80, 85, 91-92, 125
Glutinous rice flour: 19
Grapefruit meat: 88-89

J
Jackfruit: 16, 86, 95-96, 128, 138-139

K
Kappa carrageenan: 17, 46, 48, 53, 69, 103, 133
Katsu: 56
Kelp: 23, 149, 151, 153, 157-159
King oyster mushrooms: 53, 143
Konjac gum: 17, 69, 108, 158

L
Lactic acid: 23
Lentils: 39
Lion's mane: 14, 58-59, 159
Liquid smoke: 25, 39, 41, 45, 48, 52-53, 57, 67, 121, 125, 127, 129, 131, 137, 143, 153
Lobster: 14-15
Lobster mushroom: 14-15
Lox: 153-154

M
Marbled seitan: 46
Marmite: 23, 38, 40-41, 44, 46, 48, 52-53, 56, 59, 67, 91, 125, 137, 139
Meat: 10-12, 14, 17, 19, 22, 24-25, 28, 30-32, 34-35, 44, 46, 48, 52, 56, 58, 62, 66, 68-69, 72, 80, 84-85, 88-89, 100, 118, 124-126, 128, 130-131, 133, 137-139, 159
Methylcellulose: 17, 30-31, 40-41, 48, 53, 85, 91, 93, 96, 111, 137
Mochi: 19, 126

THANKS AND ACKNOWLEDGEMENTS

MONICA STONE

—

This book is dedicated to you, but you still need an extra thanks for the photography, clarity, taste tester, and for being my fiancée that has had to deal with my grumpy, stressed-out self while this whole thing came together! Love you.

COLIN WEST

—

Solaro Management—Colin, thank you so much for bringing this enormous opportunity to me and for being such a massive instrumental part of the Sauce Stache team! Thank you as always for everything you do. You help keep this dream alive and definitely help pay the bills with the work you do!

TERRY AND JANIS THOMPSON

—

Dad and Mom, thank you so much for the never-ending support, love, and kindness that has always gotten me through literally everything. Mom, thank you for sharing literally every single video and post I share on Sauce Stache over on Facebook! I love coming across those posts almost every day! Love you both so very much!

MONICA, MARK, LEAH, AND MAX

—

Sister, brother-in-law, niece, and nephew. You guys are so awesome, and I love how excited you all get for everything I do; it is so incredibly motivating. Thanks for sharing my YouTube stuff and all of your encouragement and excitement along the way! Love you all so much.

THE STONE AND PSHEDESKY FAMILY

—

Beth, Jerry, Sara, Jared, Isaac, and Leah, thank you for your constant love, support, and encouragement to write this book and all of your support for Sauce Stache! Love you all.

THE POKER GUYS

—

Andy, Joe, Ray, Aris, Rob, and Terrell—Thanks for listening to me blab on and on about YouTube, vegan food, this book, and everything else I know you all don't care that much about!

EMMA FONTANELLA

—

@Emma's Goodies—Strategy guide, creative inspiration, and friend! Thank you for motivating me to keep going and always pushing me to be a better creator. You are there every day through this journey and I wouldn't be able to do it without you!

ENZO FIORELLO

—

@Son of a Pizza Man—Sauce Stache Logo graphic designer, Beaker in Pot graphic designer, Tomato DNA graphic designer. Thank you, Enzo, for taking my incredibly rough visual idea of Sauce Stache and giving it an amazing look beyond what I could have ever expected.

STEVE CUSATO

—

@Not Another Cooking Show—Sounding board for recipes and inspiration. Steve, thanks for the help and laughs, man. I've been able to talk to you many times through this book journey and you've smashed creative walls many times for me! Thank you!

Hugo Villabona and everyone at Mango Publishing for believing that I could write this book!

The vegan and plant-based community for accepting me so kindly into your world!

Let's keep working on making plant-based meats even better for more and more people to enjoy.

And *everyone* that supports me over at my Patreon! Patreon.com/SauceStache

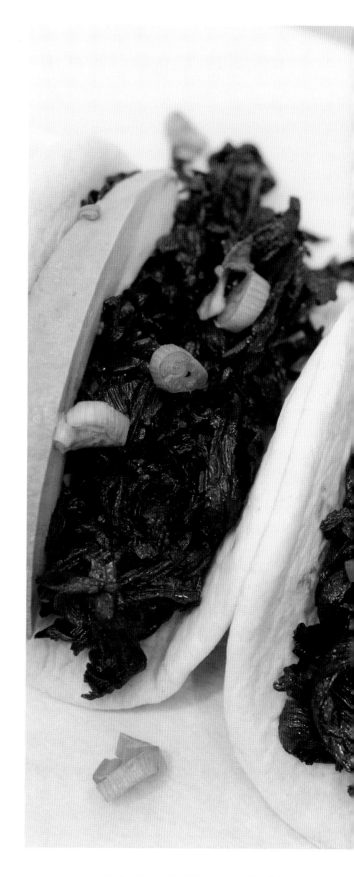

ABOUT THE AUTHOR

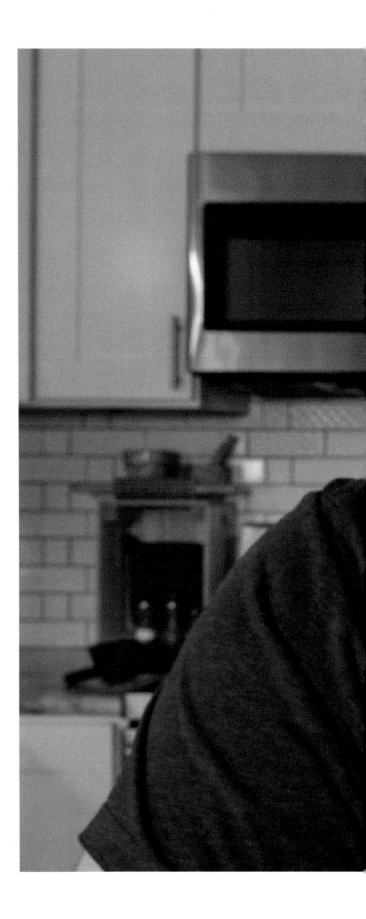

Mark Thompson grew up an avowed AV nerd and food lover in Ohio, where he split his time in the kitchen between learning to cook and taking apart small kitchen appliances. He spent most of his career in IT before founding the Sauce Stache YouTube channel in 2016. His work combines his enthusiasm for technical deconstruction with a passion for creating accessible yet impressive plant-based dishes. Although not a trained chef, Mark's work combines equal parts classic technique, engaging banter, and molecular gastronomy to charm viewers and challenge them to cook outside their comfort zone. Vegan and vegetarian food doesn't have to be boring. Mark's innovative approach to treating recipe development like the weirdest, most fun science experiment in the world is proof that a plant-based diet truly can contain multitudes of delicious options.

In just four years, Mark's content has garnered more than nineteen million cumulative views on Facebook and YouTube. In 2018, he made the move to creating content for Sauce Stache full time, and he's excited to take the brand to the next level. Mark currently resides in Florida, where he shares a home-turned-urban jungle with his fiancée and his dog.

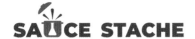

YouTube.com/saucestache
Facebook.com/saucestache
Instagram.com/thesaucestacheguy
Twitter.com.saucestache
Saucestache.com

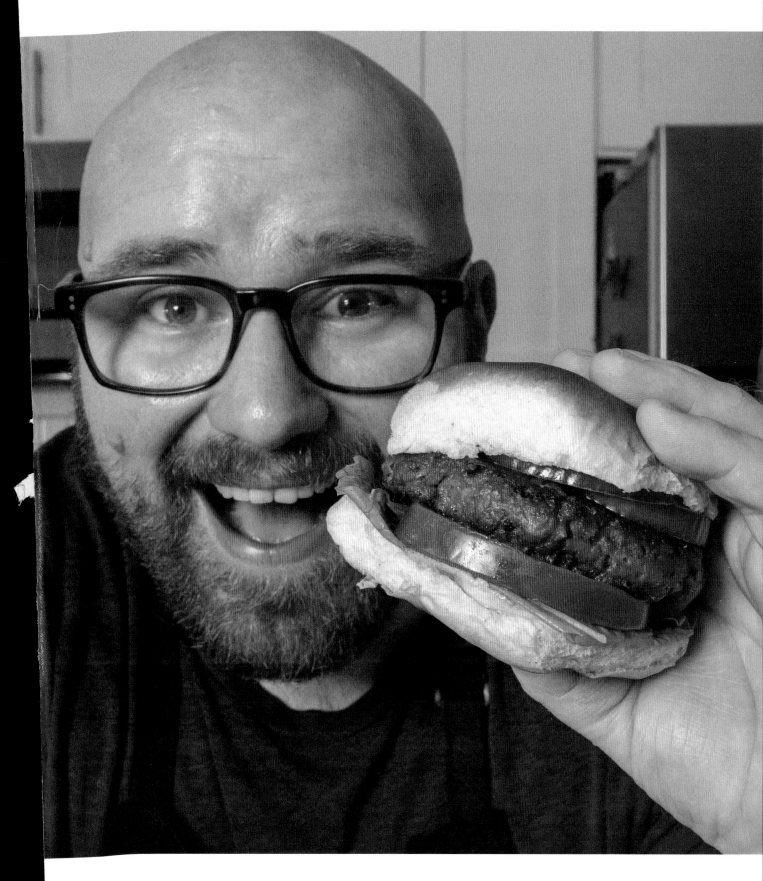

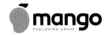